Disability Services and Disability Studies in Higher Education

Other Palgrave Pivot titles

Erika Mansnerus: **Modelling in Public Health Research: How Mathematical Techniques Keep Us Healthy**

William Forbes and Lynn Hodgkinson: **Corporate Governance in the United Kingdom: Past, Present and Future**

Michela Magliacani: **Managing Cultural Heritage: Ecomuseums, Community Governance and Social Accountability**

Sara Hsu and Nathan Perry: **Lessons in Sustainable Development from Malaysia and Indonesia**

Ted Newell: **Five Paradigms for Education: Foundational Views and Key Issues**

Sophie Body-Gendrot and Catherine Wihtol de Wenden: **Policing the Inner City in France, Britain, and the US**

William Sims Bainbridge: **An Information Technology Surrogate for Religion: The Veneration of Deceased Family in Online Games**

Anthony Ridge-Newman: **Cameron's Conservatives and the Internet: Change, Culture and Cyber Toryism**

Ian Budge and Sarah Birch: **National Policy in a Global Economy: How Government Can Improve Living Standards and Balance the Books**

Barend Lutz and Pierre du Toit: **Defining Democracy in a Digital Age: Political Support on Social Media**

Assaf Razin and Efraim Sadka: **Migration States and Welfare States: Why Is America Different from Europe?**

Conra D. Gist: **Preparing Teachers of Color to Teach: Culturally Responsive Teacher Education in Theory and Practice**

David Baker: **Police, Picket-Lines and Fatalities: Lessons from the Past**

Lassi Heininen (editor): **Security and Sovereignty in the North Atlantic**

Steve Coulter: **New Labour Policy, Industrial Relations and the Trade Unions**

Ayman A. El-Desouky: **The Intellectual and the People in Egyptian Literature and Culture: Amāra and the 2011 Revolution**

William Van Lear: **The Social Effects of Economic Thinking**

Mark E. Schaefer and John G. Poffenbarger: **The Formation of the BRICS and Its Implication for the United States: Emerging Together**

Donatella Padua: **John Maynard Keynes and the Economy of Trust: The Relevance of the Keynesian Social Thought in a Global Society**

Davinia Thornley: **Cinema, Cross-Cultural Collaboration, and Criticism: Filming on an Uneven Field**

Lou Agosta: **A Rumor of Empathy: Rewriting Empathy in the Context of Philosophy**

Tom Watson (editor): **Middle Eastern and African Perspectives on the Development of Public Relations: Other Voices**

Adebusuyi Isaac Adeniran: **Migration and Regional Integration in West Africa: A Borderless ECOWAS**

palgrave▸pivot

Disability Services and Disability Studies in Higher Education: History, Contexts, and Social Impacts

Christy M. Oslund
Coordinator of Student Disability Services, Michigan Technological University, USA

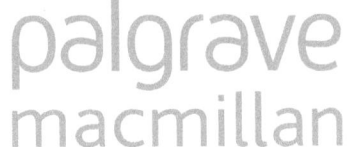

DISABILITY SERVICES AND DISABILITY STUDIES IN HIGHER EDUCATION
Copyright © Christy M. Oslund, 2015.

All rights reserved.

First published in 2015 by
PALGRAVE MACMILLAN®
in the United States—a division of St. Martin's Press LLC,
175 Fifth Avenue, New York, NY 10010.

Where this book is distributed in the UK, Europe and the rest of the world, this is by Palgrave Macmillan, a division of Macmillan Publishers Limited, registered in England, company number 785998, of Houndmills, Basingstoke, Hampshire RG21 6XS.

Palgrave Macmillan is the global academic imprint of the above companies and has companies and representatives throughout the world.

Palgrave® and Macmillan® are registered trademarks in the United States, the United Kingdom, Europe and other countries.

ISBN: 978-1-137-50245-2 EPUB
ISBN: 978-1-137-50244-5 PDF
ISBN: 978-1-137-50243-8 Hardback

Library of Congress Cataloging-in-Publication Data is available from the Library of Congress.

A catalogue record of the book is available from the British Library.

First edition: 2015

www.palgrave.com/pivot

DOI: 10.1057/9781137502445

This book is dedicated to my parents, Dick and Karen Oslund, who believed in my potential when common sense and standardized tests suggested they didn't have much to work with. Thank you for the support, love, and dedication you have shown; you provided the foundation upon which I have built.

Contents

Introduction		1
1	The Campus Divide: Teacher or Service Provider	7
2	Religious Texts and Popular Media	20
3	Logic, Law, and the Fight for Education	37
4	Disability Services and Higher Education	52
5	Disability Studies and Higher Education	70
6	Barriers to Interactions between Disability Studies and Disability Services	83
7	Potential Impact of Intentional Interaction and Coalition Forming	94
8	Building Collaborative Efforts through Coalitions	104
Works Cited		117
Index		123

Introduction

Oslund, Christy M. *Disability Services and Disability Studies in Higher Education: History, Contexts, and Social Impacts*. New York: Palgrave MacMillan, 2015.
DOI: 10.1057/9781137502445.0002.

Talking about disability is difficult. Even understanding all the layers that complicate the conversation requires some analysis. What follows is a less than an exhaustive list, just some select examples of issues which nuance the discussion and understanding of disability.

Let's start by thinking about how we each, as individuals, are positioned in relation to disability. Some who read this will be disabled, some will not; some will consider themselves disabled, others will not; some would be considered disabled by other members of society but might not think of themselves as disabled; some might consider themselves disabled but their community might dispute this identity. As you the reader approach the topic of disability, how do you identify yourself? How do you think your society would identify you? Do these identities match? How might it impact you if they do not match, that is, if you see yourself one way and your society would suppose a different identity for you? Throughout what follows I will on occasion ask the reader to pause and think about their own relationship, thoughts, and experiences with the topic at hand.

I will use myself as an example of the complicated nature of identity within society and identity within an individual when it comes to disability. I live with disabilities. Not everyone who meets me realizes this. In part, what they recognize about the nature of my disability depends on the circumstances under which they encounter me, their experience with and understanding of disability, their own identity and what they may identify as a disability. If a person encounters me over the phone they will have one impression of me; if we have a physical meeting they will form another impression of me. Even the type of day I'm having (I have a condition which causes my mobility to fluctuate) will affect whether another is likely to think of me as disabled or not. There are further complications: I also live with a disability which impacts my capacity for language processing, including my competency as a speaker, reader, and writer. If someone meets me when I am tired and having trouble finding the right word to use or if I take part in written communication at a less than optimum moment (email isn't always my friend) then I leave a different impression with people than when I am able to take my time to review what I have said or written and to revise my words. I often feel that I struggle to adequately express my ideas, even though I know my communication benefits from many years of practice and sometimes from the additional assistance of editors and proofreaders. I also recognize that feeling disabled varies from day to day. While some of it depends on the circumstances surrounding me, such as the accessibility of spaces and interactions with others who are more/less aware of disability, some also depends on how I'm feeling physically and how impaired my mobility is in circumstances where I'd like to be able to do more than I am able to in a given moment. In other words, not only is my identity within society complicated, but also my personal identity is complicated.

Identity is so complex that it inspires work in many fields of study, including work related to identity and disability. Yet, identity is only part of what complicates conversations about disability. Another impediment to clear communication when we discuss disability comes from language itself, or the words we use to discuss disability. Are the disabled a community? From a legal standpoint, for example, "the disabled" are a protected group under specific situations and what those situations are can vary from country to country. Tobin Siebers postulates that disability is a "cultural and minority identity" (2008, p. 4). However, it is also argued that people with disability are too diverse to be considered one community and to consider all disabled a single community would be like considering all minority communities a single community; while there may be some overlap in experience that two individuals would share, there are also many differences in the kinds of experiences we have based on a range of factors including socio-economic background, gender, sexual identity, education, what type and number of disabilities an individual lives with, and so on.

The words groups use to identify themselves, or that are used to identify them, also vary between nations. As a British editor that I once worked with pointed out to me, while those within North America used the term Little People, this was not a universal term. Currently in the UK the National Health Service (NHS) refers to "Restricted Growth (dwarfism)"; there are both a Restricted Growth Association and a Little People UK association, demonstrating that among those living with restricted growth there is also some difference of opinion about the preferred terminology to be used. This is an example of another language complication: how does one respectfully speak about the way contexts might impact some people while: (a) speaking to an audience that has the potential to be in different nations and (b) recognizing that there is often no one mutually acceptable term used for referencing groups? And if one never speaks of those who would be within a group because one does not wish to use any label/name then is one in effect erasing the existence and realities that specific groups of people are faced with? Are we denying people's existence by never speaking of them or just ignoring social contexts which may be particularly impactful on specific groups in specific contexts?

Language contains many nuances. Should we refer to "people with disabilities" or "disabled people"? Neither of these terms is universally accepted. As Mallett and Slater explain, in the UK, the term "disabled people" was chosen by activists; their goal was to "shift disability from a medicalized 'problem' residing *within* an individual, to a 'problem' of social inequality" (p. 91). In many other contexts, including Canada, the U.S. and the World Health Organization (WHO) the term "people with disabilities" is used; as WHO has written, "disabilities is an umbrella term" referencing that physical and social contexts as well as a person's own body may all contribute to the level of "impairment" preventing full inclusion/participation that a person may experience (p. 92). Both terms were carefully chosen and have philosophies of personhood behind them, which someone new to contexts where the terms are used will often not be aware of.

I personally tend to self-identify as a disabled person, not a person with disabilities. I do not think there should be a stigma in this identity (being a disabled person) any more than there should be a stigma attached to my eye color, that is, they are both realities that are part of what I live with. As Mallett and Slater also point out, there is a segment of the community that self-identifies as disabled who, following the example of Queer Theory are positing the possibility of Crip Theory. This will be discussed in more detail in what follows.

For some of us though, it is less a matter of feeling we are proponents of Crip Theory and more a matter of recognizing that even when all social contexts have been stripped away, our own physical embodiment remains a challenge. Tom Shakespeare's observation that there was a point in life where, "I experienced my increased disability as resulting more from my own lack of functioning than as a result of inaccessible environments, although of course I have experienced my share of those" (2013, p. 6). In other words, for some of us our lived experience is that disability isn't just out there—in our society or the inaccessibility of spaces or opportunities—it is also within our own bodies which on some days are wracked in pain or simply not able to do what we would ask of them.

Personally, I find my identity and language have been influenced by my background, including growing up in the midst of others with disabilities, my education which unfortunately did not benefit from courses in disabilities studies and which has been influenced by Canadian-British culture, and I have come to the conversation in disability studies as a mature person who has spent years entrenched in the many details that created my world view. I remain torn about how to use language related to disabilities and I recognize that it is different when I speak of myself than when I speak of others, particularly when my "speaking" is in a written format that can be taken into contexts that I cannot foresee.

I do not speak on behalf of all people who self-identify as disabled, and how I choose to speak of myself may not be how another person may choose to speak of either him or herself—or theirself—if we're trying to include language which includes people who prefer gender-neutral language. It is also important to realize that people are often labeled as "disabled" when others decide that some physical reality that one lives with is not as desirable as other physical realities. What it means to be disabled is entrenched in every society—what different groups would label "disabled" has varied through time and culture. Those of us growing up with the label of disability did not necessarily choose that label, it is an identity at least in part posited on us by our social group. I am a disabled person, in part, *not* because I chose this identity, but because the society in which I was born and raised labels the set of circumstances I live with as less advantageous than what is considered "optimum." Additionally, because people who also live with the set of physical realities that I live with have not traditionally been those who have had the power to establish or design the dominant power structures, the design of my education, work, and community were not made to automatically include me, which in turn automatically excludes me.

Education, nation of birth/upbringing, and theoretical models are all among the things that affect how one views disability, the position of social groups, the responses of communities, and the interactions of individuals. The more I think about it in fact, the more presumptuous it appears to be to try and say much about the topic of disability at all. And yet, as an educator, I know that it is only when we dare to speak with imperfect words that we can begin to have any conversation; conversations regarding disability are necessary for multiple reasons, which will hopefully become clearer as one proceeds through this work.

The focus in what follows is to try and consider how two fields [disability studies and disability services], both of which are present within institutions of higher education [colleges, universities] impact: Each other; the larger societies in which they are located; students who encounter the respective fields; and those who either would self-identify as disabled or would have an identity of disability posited on them by the society in which they live. In order to step into this conversation, however, I will begin with a broader view of how disability has been positioned in northern societies. I argue that northern social views regarding which conditions are labeled disabling have been impacted by foundational stories, ideologies, and worldviews. This dominant social view in turn impacts how those who have been viewed as disabled are not only seen but additionally impacts how we sometimes see ourselves, our potential roles, and our futures.

The very nature of what one dares to hope or dream can be heavily impacted when one lives with the identity of being "limited" due to disability. However, there is also growing push back from many who self-identify as disabled. Living with disabilities, we would argue, is not in and of itself problematic; what others decide should be our limitations is however, very problematic, as are contexts which were not designed to include us. Inclusion is a concept which continues to require readdressing as we learn more about how/when we have—sometimes intentionally, sometimes unintentionally—excluded some people in our designs. I would also argue that we do not just "design" spaces, we also design processes, groups, power relationships, and sometimes identities. Our redesigns can also prove to be flawed and tend to require regular updating. *Redesigning is a never ending process.*

In discussing disability we enter a conversation that is already in progress and one that will continue long after we have left the room. Ideally, we strive to hear each other despite the inevitable complexities that are inherent in the conversation. Unfortunately, meaning cannot always transcend how we say what we say. Responses, rewordings, and ongoing dialogue are a necessary part of reaching a place where we come closer to understanding another person's point of view or another individual's experience. I am privileged to be allowed a voice in the growing discussion about disability.

1
The Campus Divide: Teacher or Service Provider

Abstract: *Introduces the two fields being discussed, Disability Studies and Disability Services, and shows how they are tied to the respective work of two employee groups on campus: Faculty, who teach, and staff, who provide student services. Establishes why it is natural that the fields have worked independently of each other; the obstacles inherent in the working/professional environment; some of the obstacles that stand between greater collaboration between the fields. Foregrounds the idea that generations of social practices and beliefs both necessitated the development of each field and led to them being two distinct fields.*

Keywords: Disability Studies; Disability Services; faculty and staff work divide

Oslund, Christy M. *Disability Services and Disability Studies in Higher Education: History, Contexts, and Social Impacts.* New York: Palgrave Macmillan, 2015.
DOI: 10.1057/9781137502445.0003.

Conversations with people outside an academic setting have led me to think that those who do not work in academics often perceive colleges and universities as monolithic entities where everyone takes summers off from work, everyone works modest hours, and all employees know each other because, after all, the environment is like a small town. Those of us who work for colleges and universities would counter that we work long hours, we are hard pressed to find as much time as we would like for family and outside interests, and we are most likely to know the people in our immediate department; even when we are familiar with a person's name, we might not recognize that person if we saw them in the flesh. While some realities of campus life are thus obvious to those of us who work on campus, these realities might come as a surprise to those who work in different environments.

There is a basic divide in campus life between two broad divisions of employees who work in academics. On the one side of this divide are the people responsible for classroom content, teaching, and research; in North America we broadly refer to these people as "faculty" and this division includes professors, lecturers, research assistants, teaching assistants, and laboratory assistants. On the other side are the people responsible for providing student services and administration that runs the business of the university; in North America we call these people the "staff." While theoretically we all work toward the same goal—educating students—our roles, our reporting structure, our salary scale, and how our contributions are measured are perhaps surprisingly different on each side of that divide. I refer to this as a divide purposely, to create a mental image in the reader's mind of a clear division that is not regularly or quickly breeched.

Disability Studies, as a field, is primarily made up of those who would fall within the division of what I will call *faculty*, that is, they are primarily people who teach and are responsible for classroom content. *Disability Services*, as a field, is primarily made up of those who would fall within the division of what I will call *staff*, that is, they are primarily people who provide academic support services for students. For the sake of brevity then, I will refer to the different groups as faculty and staff and this reference is meant to indicate these two different types of work, as well as the different ways that this work is typically valued by an individual's employer. I recognize that teaching structures are different in different nations; however, I would argue that the reality remains that if one is primarily responsible for research or teaching, one's professional value is tied to journal publications, presentations, and *some measure of peer review from outside one's home institution*. If one is primarily responsible for academic support services however, one's value is measured differently by one's employer and more likely to be tied to reviews that give more weight to work done *within the institution*, with less weight given to still valued outcomes such as publications.

Although titles and references between countries thus might vary, the basic reality remains that the work worlds of those responsible for academic support, versus those responsible for teaching and research, have less overlap than might be imagined by outsiders to academic institutions. It is helpful to understand this in order to understand that there are also two separate worlds related to disability, disability rights, and students with disabilities when it comes to campus life, study, and activism: Disability Services and Disability Studies have developed as separate fields for practical reasons related to this naturally occurring work divide that was already present on campuses when the fields emerged and developed.

I have participated in both these work-worlds as faculty and staff. I taught at a series of three universities before switching to the staff side of life where my primary responsibilities became academic support services; it still sometimes becomes noteworthy to me how these worlds are like right and left hands, largely unaware at moments of what the other is doing, yet also capable of moments of cooperative work.

Faculty

Recognizing that there are international differences in the layers and duties of those whom I am referring to as "faculty," at this point I would focus in on those who have set the goal of obtaining a doctoral degree and spending at least part of their career passing knowledge on to students. Generally, these are the academics who share the goal of becoming tenured professors, regardless of the country they work in or the title they hold.

In order for this level of "faculty" to begin their professional career they will have completed studies at a bachelorette, perhaps masters, and eventually doctorate level; they have usually spent at least seven and often 10–12 years *preparing* to begin the process of becoming a tenured professor. The competition for entry-level positions, though it varies by field of study, is generally speaking, fierce. Having spent all those years preparing, a person then finds herself starting over, as a "candidate" for jobs. There can be 40–400 applicants with similar educations applying for an open job. The reality is, even with a PhD and years of preparation, not all job candidates will be offered a tenure-track job the first year they apply for positions. It is not uncommon for candidates to find themselves taking one year appointments which will not lead directly to a tenure-track placement. This can mean a person finds himself being stuck in a "candidate" position for several years or longer, constantly applying during the annual cycle of job hires, hoping to break into a tenure-track placement. One can read any issue of *The Chronicle*[1] to quickly realize that not all people who make it through the educational process will be offered a tenure-track job.

If one does obtain a tenure-track position there will be a sense of being a first year student all over again. *Freshman professors* are expected to immediately begin developing academic credentials which include working toward publishing journal articles, and they are expected to start serving on committees that support their department, and their university; they bear a lot of the professorial grunt work of their department as they "prove" their worth. There is an expectation that one will attend conferences of note within one's field of study, and make presentations both at conferences and within one's own institution. In Canada and the U.S., it usually requires about five years of this breakneck work-pace before a professor is ready to apply to move from the assistant to the associate level. The application process itself will require an incredible amount of work putting together binders that show one's teaching philosophy, service to their field, service to the university, and service to the larger community. If one has teaching responsibility then samples of their syllabi and assignments usually need to be presented; publications and professional awards must be listed; references from within and outside one's field/institution will have to be collected. After an assessment of all this material the candidate will either be promoted (in the U.S. and Canada the next career level is Associate Professor) or the candidate will basically want to start looking for another university where they are more likely to be able to further their career. This can be another point at which an academic career stalls or dies. If one is doing the math—by this point the academic has usually given 15+ years of their life to their studies and academic pursuits.

In order to be considered viable in one's field there are basically two ways that an academic can make the cut. A person can either be a good teacher in an institution that values teaching, or one can be a researcher/writer in an institution that values research/writing. At research-focused institutions one proves their merit by having their work published by peer-reviewed journals. On average a person needs at least five publication credits that "count" in order to make the cut to be promoted; additionally, increasingly often one will need to publish a book (with a national press, often a university press) to be seriously considered worthy of full professorship. Alternatively, one can be a successful grant or research writer, who brings significant research funding into the university and has their research published in peer-reviewed journals.

Remember, while all this research, writing, and committee work is going on there may also be teaching assignments, which include preparation, delivery, and grading. Even if one has a teaching assistant, teaching is time and energy consuming. If additionally, one works at an institution which offers graduate degrees then by the time one becomes an associate professor they will be expected to add supervising the research and writing of graduate students to their workload.

At those institutions where graduate degrees are offered, supervising successful graduate students is another element that is expected of faculty. And this is another point at which an academic's career can stall-out; usually by now a person has 20+ years in academics, from the time they have started their undergraduate work down the path to becoming a tenured professor. It is easy to imagine that to discover at this point that tenured professorship will not become a reality for one tends to be bitterly disappointing. It also tends to be a bit late to reconsider one's career goals, although of course leaving the academic life does happen. When one has spent that long in the halls of academia though, it can be difficult to feel at-home anywhere else. It can also be difficult to find a potential employer who will seriously consider someone that has spent so long "in their ivory-tower."

To recap then, faculty will have spent a number of years becoming more and more specialized in their area of knowledge; their ability to gain and keep a position is based heavily on the reputation they have among others in their specific field of study. Reputations are judged by references and publications; in the U.S. and Canada at least, if one is expected to teach and has yet to obtain tenure one must obtain overall positive reviews from students. For those whose primary role is not teaching, then it is more than ever a "publish or perish" world where journal articles and peer-reviewed books count—and are counted. More institutions are also considering how often what an individual has written is being quoted by other members of their field—just one more way of measuring the value of the individual within their field.

Hierarchically, faculty may have a supervisor/senior faculty person who gives them assignments, it is the Department Chair, however, who is considered the head of their unit. In Canada and the U.S., for example, the department one works for will answer to the Dean of their school, such as the Dean of Arts and Sciences. The Provost is usually responsible for overseeing requirements for all academic areas. The Provost assigns budgets to each academic school, the Dean of each school provides budgets for departments and makes decisions on funding new positions, or cutting funding to a department, and the Department Chair typically has final say on whether a job candidate put forward by a hiring committee is offered a position or not. Additionally, funding may be brought in by researchers who write successful grants, for example, the National Science Foundation in the U.S. funds a considerable amount of research (which may include multinational researchers/institutions) which in turn leads to funding that will support research assistants, lab assistants, and teaching assistants. Typically a department or faculty member that brings in outside funding will have more money to work with than will a department or faculty member that relies on budget allocations from the school.

Staff

In Canada and the U.S., staff are divided into two general groups; from what I can see these divisions take place despite one's nation, although the labels used may differ. Those I will refer to as *professional (administrative) staff* have graduate degrees which prepared them to take part in a specific field. Fields represented by professional staff will include Student Affairs, Housing and Residential Life, and Business Management, among others. The category I will refer to as *support staff* fill occupations that typically do not require degrees, although the individual within the position may or may not have a degree. These differences may also be reflected in whether one is considered to be an "hourly" employee (support) or a "salaried" employee (administrative). Support staff include customer service and facilities and ground's maintenance, to name just a few. For those in nations where these particular labels may not be used, I am differentiating between the staff who would be perceived as administrators and those that would not. In Canada and the U.S. disability support specialists would fall under the administrative staff label.

Depending on the campus, nonadministrative staff may or may not be offered opportunities for continuing education and professional development. Usually though, the focus is on training that is designed to facilitate having this level of staff do more work, with greater efficiency. While individual unions may provide some sense of job security, support staff are some of the first employees to be affected when there are budget cuts. Raises are either negotiated as part of a new contract and are therefore across the board, or an individual will typically have to go through a performance review and show they are doing work that is a significant addition to the amount/responsibility of work which is outlined in their original job description.

Professional staff are more likely to receive at least some financial support from their department to attend professional conferences in their field. As one rises up the managerial ladder there is increasing emphasis placed on the importance of providing "service" such as volunteer work or committee work, not just to the local campus and wider community, but also to the field one belongs to. Presentations at conferences often become expected. Professional staff are also expected to provide service on committees that make hiring recommendations; review policy (a constant activity); carry out assessment and accreditation work; volunteer for activities which support campus life and spirit; and volunteer in the community portraying a positive image for the campus in a wider arena. Professional staff members are expected to help bridge the gap between town and gown. As one upper-administrator on our campus is famous for saying, "This isn't a career, it's a way of life." Going above and beyond is just as expected of staff, even often administrators, as it is of junior faculty.

Staff hierarchy is organized within departments and divisions; divisions vary among campuses. Typically however, support staff are organized by seniority and work-level and the two do not necessarily match. Work-level is tied to the responsibilities that are assigned to individual positions; work-level trumps seniority. For example, imagine three people are employed in the bookstore to work under the supervision of the bookstore manager. There is a level 7 position responsible for tracking the budget and entering this information in a spread sheet, a level 6 position primarily responsible for customer service, and a level 5 position primarily responsible for stocking inventory. Regardless of the seniority of the individuals hired to perform these jobs, the hierarchy within the work environment will be based on the level of the job each individual is doing.

Professional staff hierarchy is similar, in that positions have set places within the institution. The difference is that the work done is not assigned an official "level" and instead organizational charts are used to give some idea of who answers to whom. At the top of this hierarchy is the President/Chancellor and their Vice Presidents; power works its way down through Deans, Associate/Assistant Deans, Directors, Assistant Directors/Managers, and Coordinators. One is hired into a position and in order to make a career/salary move one must change positions; professional staff may change positions within one institution or by moving among institutions. Perhaps one of the more significant differences between service and professional staff is that professional staff are more likely to move in order to further a career. Not only do service staff tend to view their work as a job versus a career, the wages paid for service work do not make it advantageous to move from one school to another unless one has additional reasons to move. For example, I had a friend who was a member of the local unionized service staff on the campus where I currently work. Not everyone in her family, however, was able to find regular employment in the area. When they moved she found herself in much the same work with a similar salary as what she had just left, so that from an employment perspective she had simply made a lateral move. The impact of moving was more familial in that the new location provided more employment opportunities for other members of her family.

In the modern economy, professional staff basically expect to change positions in order to further their career; for many this will mean moving at least several times. Unlike faculty, staff do not have a tenure system. While they will make connections within their field, when it comes to their immediate work environment and the longevity of their employment with any given institution, their position will be influenced by the politics of the specific campus. As with governments, when the leadership of a university changes it can have ripple effects among administrators. Service staff tends to ride out the waves of changes while professional staff may be encouraged to look for a more hospitable climate elsewhere.

Service staff do tend to be more mobile between jobs on campus, while professional staff tend to be mobile between campuses. Service staff merit is largely judged through performance reviews. Professional staff will be reviewed often with input sought from people beyond their immediate supervisor and department as part of the evaluation process; how staff are perceived within the institution carries weight for professional staff, in much the same way that how a faculty person is perceived by peers outside the institution matters. While all campus employees are first filtered through the Human Resource department, service staff will be hired by their supervisor. Professional staff will usually go through rounds of group interviews and be required to give a presentation, in a format that somewhat mirrors that used to choose faculty. The difference is that the opinion of people far outside the candidate's field will be sought, as it is important that a staff member be able to work with committees made up of representatives from across campus.

To carry this comparison back to the difference between the two sides of campus (what we're calling faculty and staff to indicate the kinds of work done) consider the difference in the way opinions are sought when a new hire is to be made. On the faculty side think of a specialization like the physics department—if physics is hiring a new instructor they are not likely to seek the philosophy department's input on who they hire. On the staff side of campus however, it is commonplace for representatives from a broad slice of campus to serve on hiring committees for professional staff. When I was interviewed for the position of disability service specialist (DSS) for example, the committee which interviewed me included a member of faculty, and professional staff including a representative from the graduate school, one of the academic support centers, the legal compliance office, and from first year programs among others (it was a large committee!)

Roles in relation to students

To start from the broadest view and work our way in—faculty's primary responsibilities are for educating students and creating and sharing new knowledge, while both professional and support staff are responsible for facilitating everything that makes campus life and education possible outside the classroom setting—from financial aid to academic support services. Staff may at times teach classes, just as I have taught a class since becoming a DSS—if one is considered a staff person, however, then one does not generally answer to an academic department the way a faculty person would. Faculty may fill administrative roles, most notably acting as Department Chair, that is, the Chair of a history department would have first been a tenured professor in history; while being chair of a department is an administrative role this is a hybrid-administrator, in that the individual typically remains a professor first, with administrative duties added. A faculty member can step down from being chair and return to "regular" duties as a professor. The hierarchy that an individual is primarily held responsible through is decided by whether the work they do, that is, *their employment role/classification*, is as faculty or staff. Faculty need to consider promotion and tenure; staff need to consider how their work fits in with the mission of their department and with their supervisor's interpretation of that mission.

People are generally familiar with the contexts that students and faculty encounter each other in. Classrooms, laboratories, seminars, and research tend to be the arenas where these relationships develop. The context for student and staff encounters, on the other hand, may be less familiar and can actually cover everything from recreation and counseling, to housing and conduct. Arguably, from the point of view of most modern students, anyone who is employed at the college they attend is supposed to be one of their "service employees" or there to serve them, but from an institutional viewpoint, staff serve while faculty teach and create new knowledge.

Faculty are in an excellent position to expose students to new knowledge and ideas. For those with teaching/lecture positions, their role allows them to choose readings and lead discussions which can challenge how a student has traditionally thought about disability. Based on individual specialist knowledge, disability can then be considered through the lens most familiar to the individual faculty member. Disability can thus be raised in basically any field that a faculty member is in, if that faculty member is willing and feels herself able to provide a foundation for the students in the class. Not all faculty, though, will see the inclusion of perspectives related to disability as part of their teaching mandate.

Just as not all faculty see their role in education to include discussion of disability, not all staff see their role as being directly involved with students with disabilities. Among staff the viewpoint is usually held that primary responsibility for students with disabilities remains the role of the DSS on campus. Both faculty who are not involved in disability studies and staff often prefer to defer to the DSS on campus, "Tell us what we should do" being a not uncommon, *yet often unnecessary position.* For both faculty and staff this can be a matter of wanting to follow a uniform set of policies and procedures; it then becomes the DSS' role to decide which accommodations are appropriate and provide information about the accommodations to be provided. *Universally designed education* starts from the viewpoint that by designing a class to be as accessible as possible for as wide a range of students as possible, one can create a class that is "usable" for most people, dramatically reducing the need for accommodations.

Fortunately, some faculty and staff realize that providing accommodations is often just a matter of ensuring access and opportunity. I know of faculty, for example, who will provide extended test time for any student who requests it, and other instructors who are adapting universal design methods in their classroom by, for example, designing their tests to take half of the available test time and then allowing everyone up to double time to take the test. Overall, however, there is still a climate on most campuses that reflects the attitude that disability studies and disability services are specialized fields and that "the average person" isn't qualified—or perhaps interested—in participating in either until disability somehow touches their personal life. As the disability studies area continues to expand in breadth and depth, there will be more opportunities for students to encounter disability in classes and topics that they might not have expected.

Disability services, ironically, is a field that ideally works toward its own demise. While the short-term goal of a service provider is to ensure access for students in the here and now, the long-term goal is to encourage accessibility and planning which would incorporate consideration for the widest possible group of end-users. In other words, if the campus' physical spaces, policies, and procedures are designed to include everyone, then it is no longer necessary to have a DSS facilitate access. In many respects, this is an underlying commonality shared with disability studies; if society can be educated to the point where that which is labeled disabled is no longer stigmatized or excluded, then the field of study would become primarily of historical contexts surrounding disability.

Reaching across the divide

In Chapter 7 we will look at some of the early efforts that have been made to bridge the traditional campus divide that exists between faculty in the disability studies area and staff in the disability services area, while Chapter 8 will consider how society and academics can gain by greater collaboration and discussion between these fields. To be clear, this divide as I've been calling it is a historical separation present on campuses *due to the different types of work and reporting hierarchy* that each group—those working in disability studies and those working in disabilities services—is situated in. While they will at times work together, their primary missions are perceived as being complementary but unique.

Before we reach Chapter 7, however, I think it is important to further consider how we socially and historically reached our current position in relation to disability. Both disability studies and disability services grew and developed as fields due to the historical social contexts that created a need for them—and these fields were and remain needed. One cannot understand this need however, until one understands at least a brief history of the way disability has been socially situated.

Thought points

Each chapter is going to close with points that can be used for multiple purposes: personal reflection; journaling; topic prompts for discussion; starting places for essays. The ideas and information in each chapter are starting points. Further reading and discussion has much to contribute to the ideas being raised here, as does the input of each individual reader.

Chapter 1: Thought points

- ▶ As a student did I/have I had contact with disability studies/disability services in my professional role on campus (i.e., taken a class or talked to a service specialist about accommodations)? If so, what personal observations can I make about that area's role on campus? What impression have I been left with after my personal experiences?
- ▶ I have never had contact with either disability services or disability studies on a school campus. In relation to my personal context

(personal history, age, interests, etc.) what has kept me from encountering either of these areas up until now? Is my interaction with either area likely to be different in the future (why/why not?)
▸ I think access for all people, including people with disabilities, is simply a matter of having a just society where all people are equally able to participate. When I make a list of contexts where accessibility is not currently possible, what does my list look like? How many of these inaccessible contexts are related to education; to work; to recreation?

Note

1 *The Chronicle of Higher Education* is a weekly news and job information source for university faculty and administrators, published in the U.S. and distributed throughout the U.S. and Canada.

2
Religious Texts and Popular Media

Abstract: *This chapter shows how the dominate stories, both in religious and popular contexts, led to the now present correlation between stigma and disability, so that disability has automatically became stigmatized. Provides examples of ways disability has and continues to be stigmatized including examples such as eugenics, freak shows, and reality television. It also shows the link between eugenics and practices of exclusion which led to people with disabilities not just being driven from public spaces but isolated in institutions; in doing so establishes that people with disabilities were not always precluded from "public" education.*

Keywords: commercializing disability; freak shows and reality television; Judeo-Christian tradition and disability

Oslund, Christy M. *Disability Services and Disability Studies in Higher Education: History, Contexts, and Social Impacts.* New York: Palgrave MacMillan, 2015.
DOI: 10.1057/9781137502445.0004.

A reading of Judeo-Christian texts

> [16]The LORD said to Moses, [17] "Say to Aaron: 'For the generations to come none of your descendants who has a defect may come near to offer the food of his God. [18]No man who has any defect may come near: no man who is blind or lame, disfigured or deformed; [19]no man with a crippled foot or hand, [20]or who is a hunchback or a dwarf, or who has any eye defect, or who has festering or running sores or damaged testicles. [21]No descendant of Aaron the priest who has any defect is to come near to present the food offerings to the LORD. He has a defect; he must not come near to offer the food of his God. [22]He may eat the most holy food of his God, as well as the holy food; [23]yet because of his defect, he must not go near the curtain or approach the altar, and so desecrate my sanctuary. I am the LORD, who makes them holy.'"
>
> Leviticus 21: 16–23[1]

We grow up and are influenced by shared social stories and values. Even those in modern society who have never stepped foot in a synagogue or spiritual meeting room are impacted by the traditional stories that have been told and retold in these spaces because these stories at one time reached well beyond these spaces and had great influence in the wider community. The social influence and beliefs created by shared biblically based stories continue to impact social views, just as our calendars and civic holidays continue to reflect a Judeo-Christian history.

Reading religious texts and deciding what they are saying is complicated. Hermeneutics—the study and interpretation of texts—can lead to very different understandings of what a particular verse "really says" and if one were to put two theologians in a room with a text they would walk out with at least three different possible explanations of what it means. Nonetheless, socially we tend to pull out dominate themes just as some stories appear to have main points when we read them. For example, if one reads the chapter of the Bible called Genesis, one can tell they are reading a story about how God created earth and people and animals. To be raised in a society where the story of Genesis was often referenced (as it was in northern societies for hundreds of years) is to "know" that in this story God was said to be the creator of life. In what follows I am not for a moment suggesting that the readings I am about to give are the only way to interpret specific texts. I am demonstrating that if one were raised in a society where these stories where known, read, and told (as they were for hundreds of years in northern societies) one was exposed to themes in which disability and physical difference were located within individuals as differences in need of fixing or cure, and that socially, those who were physically different were often set apart in negative ways such as in the passage from Leviticus.

While most children raised with these documents and stories were traditionally taught about a God who cared for them as a father cares for his children, those children who grew up with a visible difference were raised with a different experience; at home, in synagogue, or in church they were exposed to stories and readings such as the passage from Leviticus. Some may have heard the stories without personalizing them, but others would have received a troubling message: Even God did not necessarily accept them as they were born, the way that those who "looked normal" were accepted. Children already knew that others in their society treated them differently, often in negative ways in response to their physical difference. Unlike other disenfranchised groups such as the poor or meek, those with physical difference often could not find the same level of comfort from the scriptures. For example, early Jewish communities were taught, "At the end of every seven years you must cancel debts" (Deuteronomy 15:1) providing at least temporary relief from creditors for the poor. There is no limit or end, however, for those who lived with visible difference; short of miraculous cure they remained forever outside the scope of full acceptance within many social settings, including occupying the holiest of places in the temple and in the social worship structure.

The Hebrew Scriptures, known in the Christian tradition as the Old Testament, begins with the five books of law or the Pentateuch, that is, Genesis, Exodus, Leviticus, Numbers, and Deuteronomy. These books have an important place in both Jewish and Christian traditions. In the Jewish tradition the Pentateuch defined the relationship between God and human, telling humans what behaviors were acceptable and unacceptable. The Ten Commandments (such as "honor your father and mother") make up just a small portion of the laws. The laws also include rules for which animals were clean and unclean to eat, and how people could make themselves spiritually clean and unclean—the laws cover all aspects of life. At the time these scriptures were written, Jewish law was concerned with spiritual cleanliness and wholeness, which included not bringing that which was "blemished" before God. The Jewish people believed themselves to have a covenant—basically a legal agreement—between themselves and their deity which required them to keep God's laws and in return God would maintain the Jewish nation, in part by leading them to a "promised land." Leviticus, verse 21, passages 16 to 23, is an example of one of the laws the people believed they were responsible for keeping. The ancient Israelites understood that they were to maintain the visibly "blemished" as part of their community, allowing them a share of food to eat; however, those who were notably different were not considered whole, and therefore not able to directly approach the holiest of holy places; similarly, blemished animals were not acceptable for certain kinds of sacrifice. The people believed that only that which was unblemished was acceptable for God and visible marks disqualified animal and human for the holiest of purposes.[2]

The Aaron mentioned in Leviticus was Moses' brother and had been given the responsibility of leading the worship life of the Jewish people. Under normal circumstances the men in Aaron's family would make their living as temple priests and were the only people eligible for this job. Being a temple priest was a prestigious and honorable calling. A visibly "blemished" man, however, could not pursue the family vocation in its entirety in that he could never enter the holiest part of the temple. This would prevent such men from obtaining the socially prominent positions that their male relatives could all achieve. Leviticus is written in such a way that it sounds as if God was telling Aaron's family, "do not let the blemished come too near me."

The work you are now reading, however, is not a doctrine of faith, and I will therefore freely argue that the passage from Leviticus is a representation of what *humans thought* was expected of them; the concerns voiced are human concerns. Men worried about keeping those who looked different out of the most privileged social locations and roles. The inner temple was a location; being a priest who offered sacrifices there was a vocation. Those with visible differences were excluded from this inner sanctum and from the social esteem that accompanied the occupation. Leviticus 21 is an example of how people have historically hesitated to treat those who are considered different as part of the mainstream social group. Even when acknowledging that such men might have a place at the table, it has been maintained that they should not be treated like everyone else. Whether it was fear that visible difference was a sign of sin, a lack of cleanness, or perhaps even fear that God, like humans, would find the sight of such people disquieting, humans have a long tradition of justifying their need to set those who were visibly different apart from the mainstream. During the five years I studied at seminary, it struck me more than once that people have a habit of enshrining our own fears, prejudices, and political concerns in the words, and actions, that we attributed to our gods. In Geneses, for example, the story is told of God preferring the smell of Abel's offering of fatted meat to Cain's offering of fruit and vegetables—from the beginning we have told stories that portray gods as sharing the tastes, ideas, and prejudices of the men who were telling the stories.

Consider also that in the stories that are told about Jesus, stories related to illness and physical difference are always stories of healing and miraculous cures—there are no stories about acceptance of a person with a disability as he or she was, nor did Jesus have visibly disabled followers. I am among those who would argue such stories reflect the *political* view of the original story tellers, the view that Jesus could potentially be a leader who would mend a broken kingdom, returning the Jewish people to greater independence at a time when they lived in servitude to the Romans. As N. T. Wright (1998) points out in the foreword to the new edition of *Conflicts, Holiness, and Politics in the Teachings of Jesus*, life for the Jewish people whose faith placed them at odds with the Roman occupiers of their country was a constant intertwining of religion and politics, "Politics was based on religion; religion was necessarily expressed in terms of national life" (p. x). The implication for people hearing and reading these stories was that even Jesus appeared to work from a *medical model* of disability, seeing physical differences as a brokenness in need of fixing.[3]

> [46]Then they came to Jericho. As Jesus and his disciples, together with a large crowd, were leaving the city, a blind man, Bartimaeus (which means "son of Timaeus"), was sitting by the roadside begging. [47]When he heard that it was Jesus of Nazareth, he began to shout, "Jesus, Son of David, have mercy on me!"
>
> [48]Many rebuked him and told him to be quiet, but he shouted all the more, "Son of David, have mercy on me!"
>
> [49]Jesus stopped and said, "Call him." So they called to the blind man, "Cheer up! On your feet! He's calling you."
>
> [50]Throwing his cloak aside, he jumped to his feet and came to Jesus.
>
> [51]"What do you want me to do for you?" Jesus asked him. The blind man said, "Rabbi, I want to see."
>
> [52]"Go," said Jesus, "your faith has healed you." Immediately he received his sight and followed Jesus along the road.
>
> Mark 10: 46–52 (NIV)

The scripture writers who eventually wrote down these stories had their own agenda—portraying Jesus, not as one of many potential leaders, but as a figure foretold by Jewish tradition—a political leader descended from King David, a figure referred to as the Messiah. William L. Lane in his biblical commentary on Mark explains several important points: Mark is now generally accepted as the first or earliest scripture to be written about the life of Jesus, influencing those writers who followed him (Matthew and Luke knew the stories Mark told and thus what he wrote impacted how they told their stories); and that "Throughout his entire Gospel, Mark bears witness to the word of revelation that Jesus is the Messiah" (1974, p. 1). Mark had a point of view from which he was telling the stories he told. Mark seemed to miss the irony of portraying Jesus as someone who intentionally upset so many social expectations such as mixing with tax collectors and not observing the Sabbath, yet appearing to share the social view that physical differences needed "curing" so that all people would meet the same social norm.

Scholars such as Wright (1998) argue that this is in large part because Mark's purpose in telling stories of miraculous healing was to prove that Jesus had an intimate connection with God, that Jesus was the Messiah and that this could be evident to people of faith no matter who they were. Whether or not one agrees with Wright's reading of this passage however, one can again see the potential impact for those who grew up hearing stories in which, for whatever reason, even Jesus treated those who were physically different as needing to be "fixed."

Jesus, the same teacher who suggested that it was easier for a loaded camel to travel through a small space than for a rich man to gain access to heaven, was not *portrayed* as ever accepting what later social groups would identify as disability; this left room for later generations to read these stories as Jesus healing disability. Given the larger social messages that Jesus taught, it makes no sense that the person, or deity, behind that message would object to the presence of physical differences amongst his followers. It suited the political message of *the scripture writers* to have Jesus cure everyone who looked different; it suited the *writer's message* of Jesus as Messiah—even more so when the difference was present but would not have been apparent to anyone but a god. My larger point is not that we agree on the hermeneutics of these stories but rather, I wish to keep bringing us back to my central point; as a foundational document the scriptures were not portraying physical difference as part of the accepted mainstream. Physical difference is being portrayed for those who heard and read these stories as something that ought to be cured. We must also be mindful that the Judeo-Christian story dominated northern societies for hundreds of years and eventually all inhabitants of these lands became familiar with the stories.

As Kathy Black (1996) explains in *A Healing Homiletic: Preaching and Disability*, Mark wanted to make clear the difference that faith could make while also pointing out that the people who should have most clearly known Jesus was the Messiah—his disciples—often seemed to be oblivious to this, while people of faith were literally being cured directly in front of them.

> [25]And a woman was there who had been subject to bleeding for twelve years.
>
> [26]She had suffered a great deal under the care of many doctors and had spent all she had, yet instead of getting better she grew worse. [27]When she heard about Jesus, she came up behind him in the crowd and touched his cloak, [28]because she thought, "If I just touch his clothes, I will be healed." [29]Immediately her bleeding stopped and she felt in her body that she was freed from her suffering.
>
> [30]At once Jesus realized that power had gone out from him. He turned around in the crowd and asked, "Who touched my clothes?"
>
> [31]"You see the people crowding against you," his disciples answered, "and yet you can ask, 'Who touched me?'"
>
> [32]But Jesus kept looking around to see who had done it. [33]Then the woman, knowing what had happened to her, came and fell at his feet and, trembling with fear, told him the whole truth.
>
> [34]He said to her, "Daughter, your faith has healed you. Go in peace and be freed from your suffering."
>
> Mark 5: 25–34 (NIV)

This story raises another point which we need to consider. For those raised in communities where there was a belief in God, which again was the majority of inhabitants of northern society for generations, there was implicit in the social understanding of God that God knew human faults and failings even when they were not visible to other people. Lane states that Mark is using this story "as a call for radical faith" (1974, p. 194). This story reinforces the idea that Jesus, like his "heavenly father, God" could see that which a person could hide from all others. Is it so hard to imagine that those who could hide their differences from their fellow humans carried an emotional weight knowing that their difference was visible to God and that God might not accept them as they were, if they bore a physical difference and did not receive healing or cure?

Consider also that many people heard these stories and accepted them at face value, that is, physical differences too outside the norm ought to be cured because they were not acceptable. These differences were not being identified as problems within society [such as discrimination based on appearance] but rather as problems within individuals, problems which when possible ought to be fixed. Later, we will return to this point of making disability a problem within individuals in need of fixing—remember for later that one of the influences of this view point grows from hundreds of years of hearing and reading religious texts in such a manner that society heard these messages being reinforced.

Historical popular-cultural responses to disability

Religious texts like the Pentateuch and the New Testament are not the only social factors which influenced how physical difference was perceived by both individuals and their society. In his book *Stigma*, sociologist Erving Goffman (1986) points out that early Greeks used stigma—physical marks, *intentionally* placed on a person's body—to indicate that a person had some internal deficit that others in their society should be aware of, for example, a person could be branded a traitor or liar.[4] The person was visibly marked as a constant reminder to society that there was something morally undesirable about the individual (Goffman, 1986, p. 1). Goffman goes on to explain how this idea of the body being physically marked transitioned by the time of the Christian communities to influence language and thought. "Stigmata" in a religious sense are physical signs of the crucifixion such as spontaneous bleeding from the palms of the hands and, in many religious communities, are considered a sign of great spirituality. Stigma in a social sense, however, is negative. To be socially stigmatized is to be marked by physical difference at birth or by later accident, which from that point on visibly sets the individual apart from other members of their society, with negative overtones to this separation. To say someone is stigmatized is to say they are marked in a negative way.

Where stigma had once been intentionally inflicted by people onto those who were to be avoided due to their poor moral character, society began to treat anyone who looked different as someone who was to be avoided. Anyone who looked different was now stigmatized, considered marked by nature/God as undesirable. Goffman argues that society justifies stigmatizing those who appear different by *believing there must be a reason for that difference*, that is, either the person or one of their ancestors must have done something that lead to the person carrying their physical mark. Given that people once intentionally marked those who had been judged to be in some way deviant, and believing that our gods share our value systems, it is not hard to see how superstitious people would come to believe that God had marked certain people for some inner sin, or some sin of their ancestors. Unfortunately, while we now consider ourselves educated and informed, we continue to stigmatize people who do not fall within the range of looks that are considered part of the norm according to social standards of the time, that is, we treat them differently, we set them apart, we are less comfortable around them. There is also a social impetus to label visible differences as *disability*. *The stigma associated with difference was thus transferred to that which was labeled disability*.

This in turn led to the historical social belief that disability could be a sign of moral defect, a view which was reinforced by the social media going back hundreds of years: plays, books, and laws all reflected the bias that those who were viewed as disabled/physically different were undesirable, less intelligent, or deviant in spirit and mind as well as body. Consider Shakespeare's *Richard III* as an example, which has been popular and performed since about 1592. For Shakespeare and his audience, Richard III was a villain. In the play, Richard is portrayed as a physically twisted man whose external defect is meant to mirror his internal demonism. Shakespeare gives the opening speech to Richard and while many are familiar with the first line, "Now is the winter of our discontent" how often do we stop to think about the significance of the character, in the same speech, *describing himself* as:

> I, that am curtail'd of this fair proportion, Cheated of feature by dissembling nature, Deformed, unfinish'd, sent before my time Into this breathing world, scarce half made up, And that so lamely and unfashionable That dogs bark at me as I halt by them....

The character himself is saying that he is so awfully twisted in form and function that even beasts recognize him as stigmatized. For the purpose of our discussion it is important to note that the actual historical Richard III does not appear to have had any great physical mark, although thanks to literature from Shakespeare's time forward we tend to think of Richard as increasingly unbalanced in mind and form.[5] Following Shakespeare, a number of playwrights would portray Richard as deformed, a way of physically manifesting the evils that were read and written onto his character. In other words, he was portrayed as physically different and disabled to "show" the audience that he had moral defects; popular media began to use the act of physically disabling a character as a plot device to indicate to the audience that the person was morally suspect.

Richard's portrayal in the popular media as a lame hunchback who was sinister, is one example of how "disabling" someone could be used as a character device to intentionally stigmatize them. Imagine the impact on people in society who were also labeled disabled or who were physically different, when for hundreds of years the portrayal of disability is negative. Unfortunately, this disabling-to-stigmatize a character became a popular literary device.

In the dichotomy where disabled meant morally suspect and ablebodiedness seemed to be a precursor for being/becoming morally whole we can begin to understand why even the disabled themselves felt a need for a cure or miracle as part of seeking admittance into mainstream society. When we begin to understand how historically there has been an intertwining of the social suspicion that physical difference was viewed as a possible indicator of moral flaw we can begin to understand why generations of people have sought miracle-cures. For some, cure was a release from pain and suffering; I would suggest however, that miracles and cures have also been sought as those who have been stigmatized try to have their mark removed so that society will no longer treat them as suspect. Seeking a "cure" has lead countless people to travel to holy sites where miracles are said to take place, or to pray to saints who are purported to have facilitated miraculous cures. Religious icons became business, a business which continues to this day. My local grocer, for example, is one of many who has a shelf stocked with saint candles. Each candle carries an image of a religious figure and notation of the causes that the saint can help with, such as curing illness. Those who have strong enough faith, pray faithfully, and are found spiritually worthy, continue to be told that miracles are possible.

Ironically, the same people who were thought to have been marked due to sin, were, in the case of miraculous cure, now expected to show such great purity and faith that God would remove the mark from their body. We must be mindful that this is a social expectation—fellow members of society held the belief that the "pure and righteous" would be granted miracles. When an individual was not cured, they themselves were blamed by their society— their faith was not strong enough and thus they had been found unworthy. This message that difference is an individual problem needing fixing continued to be socially reinforced. Within their social groups, and using their authoritative sources of religious texts and common knowledge influenced by popular media, the public believed that great purity and faith would result in the righteous person being "healed." Nor have such ideas died out.

I recently encountered a web site whose writer was addressing the reasons that miracle-cures are no longer so commonplace. The number one reason this web-writer offers for miracle-failure is lack of faith. In Biblical times faith was primarily required of the person seeking healing, in modern times it is also required of those who pray for the miracle. The would-be *healer's* faith must be unwavering. This web-writer warns that too often faith-healers are only hopeful, not unshakable in their conviction that a miracle is warranted. In modern times it has become necessary for both healer and the miracle seeker to have faith that is "strong enough." What has not changed is the underlying message that miracles only happen for those who are worthy and, therefore, a lack of miracle is due to human failings. The implication remains that those who are not "cured" are in one way or another still individuals with problems that need fixing. The focus remains on the person, not on society or the social practices which isolate and marginalize people because they have a physical difference. By the time Disability Studies developed part of the work members of the field would face would be the uphill battle of convincing larger society that being physically different does not automatically equate to an individual needing to be cured or "fixed."

Freak shows

Perhaps the most contentious place popular culture and physical difference intersect would have to be the freak show. Freak shows were part of the world of carnivals, with the height of their popularity occurring from the 1840s to the 1940s in the U.S., although shows, particularly those owned by P. T. Barnum, did tour internationally (Bogdan). In his book *Freak Show: Presenting Human Oddities for Entertainment and Profit*, Robert Bogdan explains that he began researching freak shows as part of his research on social presentations of disability and the disabled (Bogdan, 1990). What he found, however, was more complex than he expected. While the world of carnival side shows did make exhibits of those who were different—not just those labeled disabled but also those from diverse cultural backgrounds, and those with "odd" talents like sword swallowing—the shows also provided work and community for people who otherwise might have remained isolated and in poverty. There was certainly exploitation, however, there are also cases of side show "freaks" who became wealthy and/or celebrities, like Tom Thumb (Charles Stratton) or Chang and Eng the conjoined twins. Others, like men and women born without arms or legs, were able to earn a living exhibiting themselves, at a time when people were often forced to beg in the streets to feed themselves. While the members of a freak show were still stigmatized in the wider world, the side show allowed them an opportunity to work, make friends, and play a role in creating identities which they could choose to market for their living. While the sideshow was not a utopian world, it provided an alternate option to begging and relying on both institutionalized and informal charity.

One can argue that reality television has become the newest makeover of the freak show. Television shows have followed conjoined twins, the morbidly obese, children with progeria, people with unusual skin conditions etc. Similar to freak shows of the 20th century, which incorporated "scientific" information into the pamphlets that also featured mainly fictitious life stories of those being viewed, reality television usually adopts a "documentary" tone when following those who are visually different. Those of us who watch these shows can assure ourselves, we are not staring just because these people look different, we are watching because this is an educational context and we are learning more about the lives others lead and the challenges they face. Those who choose to be portrayed have an opportunity to take part—at least to a limited degree—in how their story is told, and may obtain some financial return for allowing people to look. Some participants also say they wish to inform others about what their life is "really" like. Additionally, there is a degree of celebrity which can be attached to becoming popular as the result of a reality show; personal speaking engagements have followed for some reality show participants, as have opportunities for further television work.

What is perhaps most significant though, is that while our society now takes a dim view of the historical freak show—Bogdan writes that he has felt a need at times to justify the connection in his studies between freak shows and disability—socially we have found other ways to hold the visibly different up to be watched. How we watch them has changed. We no longer have to physically be present in the same room, we can quietly stare from the spaces of our own homes. And this staring continues to be a double edged sword; we objectify others at the same time that we help create their celebrity and increase their finances. Some people decry this as exploitation, but just as in the case of earlier freak shows, capitalism has a place for people marketing themselves for their own purposes, just as some will continue to be marketed by others for the gain of others.

Legal response to disability

While freak shows became popular in the 1840s, by 1867 San Francisco had passed the earliest of what Susan Schweik (2009) refers to as the "ugly laws." These laws, which were passed in many cities and towns in the years to follow, were attempts to make illegal the activity of public begging, thus removing from public view the "unsightly" beggars who were thought to be "blighting" the streets. Many of those trying to survive through begging had disabilities, including veterans of the Civil War, people who had been disabled during the California Gold Rush, as well as the traditional beggars—those who had been born with a physical disability, those who were being maimed in increasing numbers by industrialization, and the mentally ill. The main alternative to begging for survival were poorhouses or workhouses; some churches also continued to provide almshouses—almshouses being a tradition that has roots in early monastic times. It was expected that family and church would help those who could not work or could not find employment, while those who had no support network or whose needs were greater being left to institutionalized poorhouses or street life begging.

The increasing implementation of laws banning public displays of physical differences, including those with disabilities, also impacted the freak show, particularly the shift from displaying "freaks" for the sake of gawking at their physical oddities, to a pretense of displaying them for medical reasons. For example, in 1903 the State of Michigan passed *Act 103* which made it illegal to display "deformed persons for profit" unless the display was for "scientific purposes" including as part of an exhibit in a "museum" (Schweik, 2009, p. 101; *Act 103*). In this, P. T. Barnum had once again shown himself a man before his time, having long sold tickets in New York to *Barnum's American Museum* where "human oddities" were among the displays (Bogdan, 1990).

These so-called ugly laws were the beginning of legalizing the removal of those with physical differences from public sites and thus from public view. Previously it had been accepted that even the marginalized had a "right" to beg and be seen and be in social spaces. As social norms shifted, the impetus grew to keep those with visible differences, including disabilities, out of sight of the rest of society by removing them from public spaces. If people were not to be seen in public, then where were they to go?

Eugenics and institutionalization

Charles Darwin's cousin, Sir Francis Galton, was the father of *eugenics*—a concept he introduced and explained in the 1883 publication, *Inquiries into Human Faculty and its Development*. Galton proposed that nature did not equally endow all people with similar potentials; while Galton clearly states humans should not be bred to a narrow type, he would insist throughout his life that some human characteristics were desirable and others were not. In the article, "Distribution of Success of Natural Ability Among the Kinsfolk of Fellows of the Royal Society" published in *Nature* in August, 1904, Galton sets out to prove that the traits for success are inherited and can be found most strongly in the bloodlines of those who are already in successful positions. This was a "scientific" way of explaining once again that those who were unsuccessful, poor, and/or born with disabilities, were genetically less desirable than those who were successful. Some family bloodlines, Galton argued, were just better for society than others.

Galton was a proponent of *positive eugenics* proposing that humanity and the human condition could be improved over time through better breeding. The other side of this—a side that those who would follow Galton and build on his work would make much of—was that the "undesirables" ought to be kept from reproducing; not only those labeled disabled, but all of the poor, alcoholic etc., whom Galton argued had little or nothing of value to add to society and who would simply further degrade society by increasing the numbers of those like themselves. Galton himself seemed most concerned with identifying the gifted families of the British nation whose reproduction had offered the most to improving society, through contributions such as science and governance.

Unfortunately, eugenics became popular and would eventually be taken in a direction that Galton could not have foreseen—Nazis eugenics—which went beyond suggesting traits were more or less desirable to attempting to destroy every human labeled "undesirable." In between Galton and the Nazis however, there was a time of social movement where particularly those labeled disabled were first discouraged, and eventually at times legally prevented from reproducing. For example, in 1912 Henry H. Goddard published his own study of how one family exemplified the inheritability of "feeble-mindedness." *The Kallikak Family* was a narrative based on Goddard's "study" of the bloodline and background of a woman who lived at the institution where he worked, the Training School for Backward and Feeble-minded Children, at Vineland, New Jersey. A eugenics argument for the inheritability of undesirable traits, Goddard's *Kallikak Family* claimed that the studies carried out through the institution were proving that feeble-mindedness ran in families, that is, it was to be found in certain bloodlines. Goddard argued that the solution to this problem was to isolate the feeble-minded in institutions, where they could be prevented from reproducing. As the eugenics movement spread, the idea of separating the feeble-minded and other undesirables from society so that they would not reproduce spread with it. Other books and pamphlets joined the eugenics genre including still available texts such as, *The Jukes* (reprinted as *The Jukes: A study in Crime, Pauperism, Disease, and Heredity*).

Not all families were necessarily willing to institutionalize their offspring, even when they shared the larger social view that their child was disabled. At the same time, there was increasing social pressure—and sometimes family concerns—that no additional burden be created by allowing such people to reproduce. In 1924 the Commonwealth of Virginia passed a law that allowed for the nonconsensual sterilization of people who were judged to have "heredity forms of insanity that are recurrent, idiocy, imbecility, feeble-mindedness, or epilepsy."[6] In 1927 the Supreme Court decided in *Buck v. Bell* that forced sterilization was not a violation of a person's constitutional rights.[7] Forced sterilization would continue, legally, for decades. In the U.S., guardians/parents can still apply to have people who have intellectual and developmental disabilities (IDD) sterilized and this topic still can be found on discussion boards online where people debate both the moral and practical concerns related to those with IDD having their own children.

Nor is the U.S. alone in allowing sterilization of those judged intellectually unfit to parent. Consider for a moment that there remains a strong social perception in northern societies that those of "low I.Q." should not have freedom of reproductive choices, yet society has not enacted laws to stop murderers, alcoholics, child abusers or any other group from reproducing, a point we will return to in Chapter 3. As Roets et al. point out, society is more comfortable imagining people with disabilities as asexual while, "Women with 'learning difficulties' are commonly perceived as 'eternal children' and 'not quite women'" (2006, p. 171). We continue to live in a paternalistic age where using coercion to sterilize women is still perceived to be justifiable. While eugenics is now widely decried as inhumane and without merit, social views also continue to be influenced by the ideas that disability is an individual problem, located within people, and can be controlled by controlling the reproduction capacity of disabled bodies.

Chapter 2: Thought points

- ▸ Do I belong to a faith tradition that has teachings or stories about disability? If so, what do the traditional stories tell me about disability; what do they tell me about those labeled disabled? How have definitions of disability changed over time and social contexts?
- ▸ What stories come to mind when I think of disability? Are these stories positive or negative? Are these stories I would want told about me? What role do I play in my personal responses to and stories about disability? Being totally silent on a subject is also a response; if I'm silent on disability what does this say to those around me?
- ▸ How do I define disability? What authoritative sources, stories, personal experiences, or other influences have affected my definition?
- ▸ Would I be interested in attending a freak show; would I be embarrassed to do so and why/why not? How are individuals and the society they live in affected when human difference is marketed as a commodity?
- ▸ Have I seen a reality television show that focuses on someone's difference or disability? What impressions did I form about the

person? Did I see commonalities between their life and my own, and if so, did this do anything to influence my perspective of what this person's life is like? Did the show increase or decrease my feelings of being different from this "other" person?
▸ What are my thoughts about sterilizing people? Do I believe that reproduction is a human right; that reproduction should be legislated; that the will of the many should outweigh the will of the few? Can I imagine what it would be like if I were judged to be unsuitable to be a parent; a citizen; a voter?

Notes

1   New International Version (NIV) translation. Copyright Biblica.
2   The Bureau of Jewish Education has made the 26 volume *Encyclopedia Judaica* available online—a valuable resource that was once primarily available in seminary libraries can now be widely read for more information about Jewish culture and practices: http://www.bjeindy.org/resources/library/encyclopediajudaica/
3   A medical model of disability posits that physical difference is illness in need of cure. A social justice model posits that what is most likely to prevent a person from living a fulfilling life are situations created by social contexts. For example, being prevented from practicing the family trade because of how one looks is a social construct, created by others, not a result of the individual's capacity to perform the necessary duties. To quote Tobin Siebers, "...disability studies defines disability not as an individual defect but as the product of social injustice, one that requires not the cure or elimination of the defective person but significant changes in the social and built environment" (2008, p. 3).
4   The brand or cut was made as part of a social judgment about the person's character given actions they had carried out. E. Goffman (1986) *Stigma: Notes on the Management of Spoiled Identify*. New York: Touchstone.
5   The Richard III Society has an online site that attempts to separate generations of fiction from historical accounts written during Richard's lifetime; they also display a facial reconstruction developed after the discovery of Richard's grave in 2012 . http://www.richardiii.net/
6   Virginia Sterilization Act of March 20, 1924.
7   *Buck v. Bell*—274 U.S. 200 (1927).

3
Logic, Law, and the Fight for Education

Abstract: *This chapter shows how prejudice toward people with intellectual and developmental disabilities was encouraged not just by how society was interpreting their religious texts but also by the growth of the Philosophies of Reason and Ethics. Descartes, Hume, and Kant have each had a lasting impact on current understanding of what it means to be a full member of society, which can be seen reflected in modern philosophical arguments made by Jeff McMahan and Peter Singer. People with disabilities thus faced an ongoing fight not just to leave institutions which segregated them, but to gain access to full educational opportunities. It also examines the development and legacy of the Special Education classroom.*

Keywords: legacy of special education; philosophy and disability; prejudice of logic

Oslund, Christy M. *Disability Services and Disability Studies in Higher Education: History, Contexts, and Social Impacts.* New York: Palgrave MacMillan, 2015.
DOI: 10.1057/9781137502445.0005.

The popularity of eugenics began to decline after World War II. Once the atrocities of the Nazi concentration camps became known, people started to understand that there was a potential slippery-slope any time one group of people began to judge the fitness of others to have what are now considered basic "human rights." Unfortunately, those people considered disabled remained a marginalized group and, as was observed in Chapter 2, one is more likely to be sterilized if one is a disabled woman than if one is a serial killer. In arguing their cases in court, those with disabilities are often required to work in cooperation with supporters considered nondisabled in order to be given due legal process. This is particularly true for those with intellectual and developmental disabilities (IDD) who face the bias of not meeting the historical concept of having a "reasonable mind."

The bias for logic and reason

Religious stories and concepts are not the only authoritative sources which have influenced the views currently held by social groups about who should have the right to reproduction and full citizenship within a community. From our constitutions to our educational systems, the influence of philosophers such as Plato, Descartes, Hume, and Kant can be found. Philosophy has a long and rich tradition. Just as with religion though, there is a bias in philosophy against those who were seen to fall outside the "norm," particularly those with IDD. In order to take part in philosophical discussions, ideas, and thought experiments—in order to count as one of the people who are capable of "thinking"—it has been expected that a person have the capacity for reasoned logic.

In *A History of Intelligence and Intellectual Disability*, C. F. Goodey (2011) points out that we should not assume that the ancient Greeks meant the same thing we do when talking about knowledge, a person's "natural" ability to know, or one's natural ability to learn. Goodey makes this clarification because so much of later philosophy builds on interpretation of what it was *thought* the Greeks were saying about what one could know and what type of people had the innate nature required to be capable of reasoned thought. I would point out that while the Greeks may have meant something different from what we currently would mean regarding kinds of knowledge, it is precisely because so much has been built on the foundations of Greek philosophy that certain of *their words* and our interpretations of meaning and applications of these words continue to affect our ideas. As Chapter 2 began to show, we continue to judge people's ability to make choices—we continue to judge their social value—based on how we have interpreted what has been passed on to us through history. We have arrived at our current beliefs and understandings of what it is to be disabled based on many factors, including the traditional philosophical understanding of reason.

Classic rhetorical appeals as developed in Greece were built on three legs: *logos, pathos,* and *ethos*. An argument, or persuasive idea, had to have logic, it had to have emotional appeal, and it had to be made by someone whose ethical standing in the community was sufficient to carry the weight of the argument. For example, someone who had been branded a traitor would not be able to make an argument for the best interest of his home city the way a war hero who had protected the city would be able to—one man's reputation would undermine the ethics, logic and emotional appeal of his message, while the other man's argument would be supported by these same elements. *Logos* and the importance of logical thinking were particularly given increasing focus by the philosophers whose work came after the Greeks, sometimes to the extent that the philosophers who followed would insist that logic could be stripped of its emotional content, a claim the Greeks would have found dubious—and illogical. It is the very nature of people to argue for, to make our best logical appeals for, the things we care most about.

It was the ability to think, or to be a being capable of realizing that one was thinking, on which Descartes (circa 1641) would rest his entire ontological argument, that is, the argument that he could know at least the most fundamental nature of being and thus the existence of God. As he famously observed, "it must finally be established that this pronouncement 'I am, I exist' is necessarily true every time I utter it or conceive it in my mind" (p. 64). More popularly translated as "I think, therefore I am" Descartes' idea was that one can be certain that in order to have a thought one must exist, an idea that continues to influence Western understanding regarding what it means to be a rational person. Social expectations of what counted as meaningful life was morphing; once philosophers had suggested that any being capable of having sensory impressions and experiences was in some way having a meaningful life, even if some lives were more significant than others. The new standard for social inclusion was becoming that one be capable of *analytical* thought to be considered a properly reasoning being. Descartes was telling us that being aware of senses (smelling, feelings of pain) was no longer enough; what made a human mind significant compared to other animal minds was the fact a reasoning human was *self-aware*.[1] Social exclusion based on a person's inability to be a person of reason was not only given a new weight, it was given a new definitive cut off point, although in practice entire classes of people and the gender of female were automatically excluded from full status of "reasoning" even though they were self-aware. Self-awareness was the first of many cut off points; other cut offs used to deny reason included being a person of color, of a lower social class—eventually everyone who was not a white male of some social standing was found in one way or another to not be capable of "full reason."

Men of reason in positions of power "realized" that they had a duty to safeguard those less capable of reasoned thought; a duty to "protect" these who were illogical and too quick to fall prey to their own emotions; a duty to monitor the un-self-aware beings with poor judgment and simple impulses. Combined with the social interpretation of the Bible, which was also being read in such a way that it was guiding these same men of power and reason to be the patriarchal-caretakers of all they found in their world, the message seemed clear to the social powers of the time. Entire classes of beings were meant to be stewarded by the best judgment of others. Of course those viewed as disabled, particularly those with IDD, were considered to lack the capacity to hold any power or influence.

Although he was a contentious figure in his own lifetime, David Hume's writing (circa 1777) on the nature of thoughts and knowledge would become increasingly significant after his death. Hume also had great impact on a contemporary philosopher who enjoyed greater popularity during their lifetimes—Immanuel Kant. Hume began his treatise, *An Enquiry Concerning Human Understanding* from a place where he did have shared ground with other philosophers and with the men of power in his time. Hume states, "Man is a reasonable being; and as such, receives from science his proper food and nourishment: But so narrow are the bounds of human understanding, that little satisfaction can be hoped for in this particular, either from the extent or security of his acquisitions" (1777, p. 3). Hume, knowing that he was about to make contentious observations and propositions regarding the nature of knowledge started with what was considered self-evident to the ruling class of his time. Those who count in any conversations of import are reasoned men who are interested in knowing more about science and the nature of being. Think about how many people in the mid-18th century that this excluded: women; the lower classes who were more interested in feeding their families than philosophy; those who lacked access to books or the ability to read; and those who had no capacity for self-analysis or the study of science. It is the particular focus on reason and logic however, that continues to push those with IDD further to the margins—even if they were male and born into powerful families, they had no place among men of reason, excluded by the social construct of what it meant to "count" in a society that valued a particular type of "logic and reason."

Consider, for example, that by 1912 George Bernard Shaw would posit that *even a poor girl*, with education and guidance provided by an upper class male, could be taught enough to pass as a member of the upper class. In the same timeframe things became even arguably worse for those with IDD as they were now targeted for large scale institutionalization. The opening of the Royal Earlswood Hospital in 1853, was just the beginning of what would become a growing trend (Goodey, 2011, p. 15). Just as Biblical teachings had kept those with visible differences from obtaining the highest social positions, philosophical teachings were helping to justify the marginalization of those who could not pass the standard of being capable of reasoned logic. Two significant sources of moral authority—Religion and Philosophy—were being interpreted by the society of the time as supporting the marginalization of those labeled disabled as something that was both necessary and desirable.

Immanuel Kant a contemporary of Hume, would have his own particular impact on the social conscious not only of his time but continuing well into modern social thought. Through his Ethics, Kant argued that morality was also an outgrowth of rationality. To be immoral was to be illogical for, "in moral concerns human reason can easily be brought to a high degree of correctness and completeness" (1785, p. 10). In many ways this is the ultimate connection being made between logic and one's capacity for moral worth—those who are not capable of logic can never be either expected, or capable of, full human merit because they cannot be *reliably* moral beings. The strict social oversight of moral men is necessary for the proper social functioning of all those incapable of morality due to their incapacity to reason. In other words, a person who on their own behalf is not capable of reason and therefore reliable morality, can be guided, trained, and reprimanded by a moral agent so that their actions will still usually fall within acceptable standards. Note the increasing social conviction that for many reasons those considered disabled ought not to be allowed to govern themselves. As was pointed out in the previous chapter, bodies that were physically different were suspect of moral flaws; minds that were different were also judged incapable of morality.

The oversight of those not capable of reason was not the focus of Kant's Ethics, however, this connection between reason and morality became one of the influences on social thought of the time. Philosophy was supporting the social view, also reinforced by the way society was reading their Bibles, that there was both a moral and God given duty for men of power and reason to "care for" those less capable of ruling their own tastes and impulses, particularly when the individual was not capable of "reasoned" thought. This was a very influential view point in part because it was adding further support to a line of thinking already popular, that is, those who had power had power for the benefit of society and with God's blessing. The impact on everyone who was not an educated, property holding male was that they were not only ordained by God to be excluded from the most prominent social positions, but also they were unsuited by their very physical nature from being morally capable of caring for themselves or being fully responsible members of society.

Unfortunately, some philosophers continue to debate what is "owed" to, or how one measures, the value of a human life when that life is being lived by someone who has IDD or is living with severe disabilities. In "The Personal is Philosophical Is Political," Eva Feder Kittay (2010) discusses her ongoing debate with fellow philosophers of note, Jeff McMahan and Peter Singer. In Kittay's words, "McMahan argues for a two-tiered morality, one for persons, and one for nonpersons." As Kittay points out, what McMahan is actually arguing is to divide people into two groups, "Persons include all human beings who function at a certain (unspecified) cognitive level...Nonpersons include all other sentient beings...In the nonperson category, he argues, we may or may not include human beings whose cognitive capacity has never developed [or will not develop]" (p. 394).

In other words, both McMahan and Singer have argued that we have no greater moral obligation to "lower order" persons than we have to other animals. Philosophers such as Singer and McMahan continue to divide people into groups based on considerations of intellect and use this separation to argue that we cannot owe anything to a "lower order" person that we would not owe to a chimp. So, for example, if you would experiment on a chimp, you should be able to experiment on a person with IDD because we cannot owe any care to the one that we do not owe to the other. While McMahan and Singer are trying to basically argue-up the ethical obligations society has to high-functioning, non-human primates (orangutans, chimps, bonobos) they do so by trying to lower the ethical standing and moral value of humans with disabilities. These philosophers argue that based on their lack of reason, some people are owed no more than would be owed to a chimp in a scientist's lab. Singer has also argued that some physical disabilities are so severe that it should be legal to kill newborn disabled babies. His most famous debate took place with advocate and lawyer Harriet McBryde Johnson (2003) who later wrote about her meeting with Singer in *The New York Times*:

> He insists that he doesn't want to kill me. He simply thinks it would have been better, all things considered, to have given my parents the option of killing the baby I once was, and to let other parents kill similar babies as they come along and thereby avoid the suffering that comes with lives like mine and satisfy the reasonable preferences of parents for a different kind of child. ("Unspeakable Conversations.")

Singer continues to argue that infanticide of the disabled should be legal. While he is certainly a contentious figure, Singer also has a very prominent platform from which to make his ideas public. As of this writing Singer holds a professorship with Princeton University in the Center for Human Value, and in The Center for Applied Philosophy and Public Ethics of the University of Melbourne.[2] While many people find his ideas abhorrent, others pay to study with him and hear him speak; he continues to be published and to be quoted by media meaning his ideas are widely circulated in social contexts, particularly when disability is being discussed.

The education of those with intellectual and developmental disabilities

According to National Archive records, what would become the Royal Earlswood Hospital began in 1847 as the "Asylum for Idiots"; in 1848 the institution took in its first 50 patients (2001, Ref. 392). Once the institution became the Royal Earlswood Hospital the average patient count was 500. The founder of the Asylum, Andrew Reed, was concerned that those with IDD—then known as Idiots—were being institutionalized with the mentally ill—then known as Lunatics. Reed thought it better that those with IDD be housed separately, and efforts be made to provide them with some kind of education or training so that they could become self-supporting. Although a range of ages were accepted to Earlswood, preference was given to children, who had the best chance of being positively impacted by early attempts at education. Patients were accepted for periods of either five years training, or for a lifetime of institutionalization. This system continued until 1948 when the government took over control of the institution and stopped accepting new patients for lifetime commitments.

While placing people in institutions for "idiots" might seem repugnant now, at the time Reed was actually very progressive. The social policy of the time was to isolate people with IDD or mental illness and basically leave them, often in deplorable conditions, in effect prisoners who would never be freed. Reed appears to have been among a small but influential group of people in northern society who were beginning to recognize that placing thousands of people in institutions and warehousing them for life was not a desirable concept. At a time and in social circumstances where intellectual disability did not just preclude one from being accepted as a full member of society but when it was commonplace to institutionalize and forget anyone with a psychological or intellectual disability, Reed and others were arguing for no longer forcing people out of public places and instead, argued that people with IDD again be treated as members of society. This was an idea which took time to spread but there were proponents of the idea in other countries, including the U.S.

Early American views

Kim E. Nielsen in *A Disability History of the United States* points out that early Americans had a significantly different view toward disability, including mental illness, than would become commonplace by the 20th century (Nielsen, 2012). Early Americans tended to focus on finding every member of society a job so that all members of society would be contributing. In Colonial America, each community was responsible for supporting the local residents who had no families able or willing to support them, if they were unable to support themselves. As a result, if a person was capable of work—intellectual or physical—then they were put to work rather than being institutionalized. Nielsen recounts the example of Samuel Coolidge, who was born in Massachusetts in the early 1700s (p. 31).

A Harvard graduate, Coolidge's mental health declined and he began relying on his community to provide shelter and sustenance. As a result, he was returned to the town of his birth, where it was expected that in order to help support himself he would do something his education had prepared him for—teaching. At times he was too ill to teach, "wandering the streets of Watertown and Cambridge half-naked, yelling profanities, and disrupting classes at his alma matter [Harvard]" (p. 32). Communities like Cambridge continued to return him to his birthplace, Watertown, which in turn, "sometimes locked him in the schoolhouse at night to make sure that he would be there to teach the next day" (p. 32). It was not until he became unable to teach and his behavior became erratic to the point that no one would board him without keeping him locked in a room, that Coolidge stopped being a working member of his community. He spent the last year of his life locked in a room and up until that point had worked when able.

Nielsen also documents that in 1849, a social development was happening which it turns out was parallel to what was happening in England with Andrew Reed's establishment of the Asylum for Idiots (pp. 71–72). American Samuel Gridley Howe had done the groundwork and research necessary to convince the government of Massachusetts to try its own experiment with educating those with IDD; in that year the Massachusetts School for Idiotic Children and Youth was opened. Unfortunately, rather than these efforts being the precursor to greater access to education, these organizations would set the stage for further institutionalization of people who would be forced out of public spaces, particularly those identified as disabled in the years to come. What had started as an impulse to educate, ended up becoming an idea co-opted by the eugenics movement, which wanted to see "undesirables" institutionalized for life precisely to keep them separated from larger society. The eugenics movement would prove socially powerful for a number of years. In some institutions, however, educational efforts continued to be made, just as in some institutions there were only attempts to warehouse people. A person's future was partially dependent on which kind of institution they ended up in—one with an educational focus or one that was strictly meant to separate them from society.

Even in those intuitions which were designed to educate, however, an educational focus was not creating an ideal environment. The larger social conviction remained that those labeled disabled were not the best judges of their personal welfare. In *Nothing About us Without Us*, James I. Charlton brings attention to one of the single greatest issue with what would become known as "Special Education," that is, education designed specifically for the disabled. While the intent was to provide more universal access to education, Special Ed became a system that was "a badge of inferiority and a rule-bound, bureaucratic process of separating and then warehousing millions of young people" (Charlton, 2000, p. 33). Charlton reports that his own interviews with those who experienced classrooms still working from the Special Ed model found "respondents indicated that they believed Special Education made them more passive and convinced them of their lot in life" (p. 33), their lot including an inability to be their own best advocates. People put through a special education process have been taught that they should limit their expectations and realize that others needed to speak on their behalf because they are not capable; those with IDD have for generations been given the social message they should not expect full social participation, a lesson which continues because society continues to act in accordance with these beliefs. This is another set of beliefs which those in the fields of disability studies and services still find and must continue to challenge.

Nielsen documents that by the end of the World War II, it had become a standard practice for families to institutionalize their children with IDD and with encouragement from doctors, to forget about them, lest they "ruin marriages and destroy the lives of other children in the household" (2012, p. 142). Yet Nielsen says, it was parents who refused to accept this social stigma, who spoke out, organized, insisting that their children were not a curse but a "gift from God" who started the crucial first movement of not just keeping children home but insisting they be allowed into the public school system (p. 143).[3] Families and those themselves labeled disabled had to together fight for the opportunity to return to public spaces they had been banned from.

The legacy of the short bus

Our societies—and this is particularly true for Americans—are very fond of Cinderella stories, where someone who has nothing rises through personal triumph to become an individual of note. As Malcolm Gladwell shows repeatedly in *Outliers: The Story of Success*, we can tell a successful individual's story in a way that makes it appear he or she has overcome great odds to single-handedly achieve success due to their own innate ability or willpower (Gladwell, 2008). Or we can step back and look at the larger social conditions, partnerships, and in some cases the impact of being in the right place at the right time which also feed into success. How people moved from institutions which warehoused them to positions of power can be a story which is also told either/both ways. There are pioneers of the disability movement who pushed themselves beyond all social expectations and fought for basic civil rights such as attending school, finding a place to live, or taking public transport. The story of Allan however, reminds me that for those of us who were children living with disabilities prior to disability law reforms, the families we were born to and their support, willingness to advocate with/for us, and their acceptance of us made perhaps the greatest single difference to the futures we could potentially have.

Allan's story is told on the U.S. Department of Education website which celebrates 25 years of the *Individuals with Disabilities Education Act* (IDEA) as amended in 1997.[4] Meant to show the difference that IDEA has made for the disabled, Allan is an iconic figure representing what fate could be for those labeled disabled in previous generations. Born in the late 1940s, Allan was left without explanation as a foundling at an institution which warehoused people with disabilities. One must infer from what is not said in this account of Allan's life, is that *Allan must have somehow looked physically different*, perhaps been part of a minority group or with some other physically visible difference. It seems unlikely that a visibly healthy, white male infant, even one left on the doorstep of a warehouse for people with disabilities, would have automatically been institutionalized. No mention is made in this telling of Allan's story of what stigmatized him according to the society he was born into.

What is told is that when he was 35, in the 1970s, Allan had become so institutionalized, that he had taken to self-harming, slapping himself in the face to the point that he was blind and had a "heavily callused face"; when for the first time, at the age of 35, Allan was finally "assessed" he was found to be "of average intelligence" (History). It is interesting to note that Allan's story is used to highlight how far education for people with disabilities has come; yet scratching beneath the surface it would appear to be a story of how visible difference somehow sentenced Allan to life in an institution. What stigma did Allan display which landed him where he was from infancy?

The self-harming behavior that Allan exhibited is not uncommon in individuals who are warehoused in institutions. Along with self-harm, those who are left with only minimum interaction also display other behaviors observed in Allan—sitting alone, rocking and humming. These behaviors are so commonplace that for some time it was believed by doctors and staff that the behavior was another part of living with an intellectual disability. Studies that began in the 1960s and continued through the 1980s would show that if some kind of stimuli and interaction was provided, the self-harming or acting out behavior exhibited by those who were institutionalized, would markedly decline (Bragg and Wagner, 1968; Horner, 1980). Horner's study, for example, showed that even "profoundly retarded" children would play with toys and interact with adults, if they were given the opportunity to do so, rather than being left alone in sterile environments. Horner also argued that providing stimuli and interaction would decrease the incident of self-harm and could be used to modify behavior.

Scientific studies, families choosing to keep children home and taking increasing steps to advocate for access to education, and the tenacious determination of people with disabilities all came together to push the social status quo of warehousing people from infancy and instead moved toward providing families with social support so that children could have access to education. Even given how hard these basic human rights had to be fought for, however, without changes in legislation they could have proved to be temporary changes. Disability Rights activists realized this and increasing public pressure was placed on lawmakers. In 1975 the U.S. Congress enacted PL 94–142—the Public Law *Education of all Handicapped Children Act* (EHA), which has been revised as the *Individuals with Disabilities Education Act* or as it is now known, IDEA; these revisions (PL 101–476) and amendments (PL 105–17) expanded services to include assisting people with disabilities transition into adult living (History). While EHA was an important first step, children with disabilities were still not being given access to the same education as other children; they were being given access to "special education."

Special Ed was being offered within public schools, as opposed to a separate institution. This change, however, still resulted in the stigmatization of children with disabilities. Separate buses or modified vans which could provide accommodations like lifts for wheel chairs, seat belts to hold children in place, and more adult supervision were often used to transport children with disabilities to school. What started as a point of access was soon turned into another marker of difference that was also stigmatizing—saying someone rode the short bus became a disparaging comment that children and even adults sometimes used to taunt each other and imply that someone was stigmatized. Currently adults in the U.S. and Canada will still sometimes disparage one another by asking, "Did you happen to ride the short bus to school?" clearly implying that to require this kind of access is to be found lacking in some significant way. Special Ed was education but it was separate and unequal education that was not meant to prepare children for college or for the same futures as their same-age peers.

Disability rights movement

Students with disabilities and their families were discovering that there was a difference between having access to Special Ed and being prepared for futures that would include college and professional careers. In *Inclusion and School Reform*, Lipsky and Gartner discuss the steps that would be necessary in order for students with disabilities to have similar education opportunities as other students (Lipsky and Gartner, 1997). When their book was first published, in 1997, the "Current System" was still largely Special Ed and separate education for students with disabilities. At that time, legal cases were forcing school systems to integrate all children into regular classrooms with the use of aids for some children (including an adult attendant) when necessary. The movement Lipsky and Gartner were documenting was the change from the practice of school districts automatically segregating children identified as disabled, to the legal provision that a school district had to prove there was a need to keep the child segregated in a Special Ed classroom. Special Ed classes were slowly being replaced by what would eventually become known as "resource rooms" which would provide specialized education or therapy for a child at select times during the school day, with the child in-class with peers the remainder of the day.

Lipsky and Gartner also mention the development of the Individual Education Plan (IEP) which the 1991 amendments to IDEA called for as "plans to be developed, with parental and student involvement, for the transition from school age programs to adult services no later than age

16" (1997, pp. 45–46). It is interesting to note that originally the IEP was meant to reduce the amount of "labeling" that was done to students and instead shift the focus to the kinds of support and practices a student would need to transition to life in society. Due to my current work I can affirm that by the time a student now arrives at college they may find it embarrassing to have it known they at one point had an IEP in high school. Anything that is originally designed to increase access to universal social rights can become stigmatized as we with disabilities tend to share the social desire to be just like everyone else, fit in, and not require anything "special." Even those of us who are disabled sometimes have yet to recognize that services which provide access to places and processes that exclude us because they were originally designed in an exclusive manner are *necessary* to transition to an inclusive society. There remains a required shift in social views and opinions about approaches to disability, inclusion, and exclusion; education is still required to help society understand where practices of exclusion still need revision to become more inclusive. This is another reason that Disability Studies is a necessary field of study.

In Chapter 4 we will consider the kinds of adjustments that became necessary at the college/university level once students who would have been precluded from attending school finally fought their way through the K-12 system and began to arrive at college/university.

Chapter 3: Thought points

- If I were alive in the 1700s and my family had their current social position would I have been a person of power and influence, a person who was considered working material but not powerful, a person who was considered to be unfit to judge my own personal best interests? Can I imagine what it would be like to be treated as childlike my entire life as far as making personal/professional/moral choices, while still being expected to feed, clothe, and house myself?
- In my personal value system what do I believe makes a human life worth living? Do these beliefs influence how I look at people who may be living a life that doesn't meet my personal standard of "worthwhile"?
- When I am discussing or debating an idea/value with others, what do I look for in their argument? How much weight do I give to

personal experience as informing a person's opinions; how much weight do I give the "logic" of their argument? Do I place emphasis on a person's capacity for reason over their story of how they experience events? What are the implications of valuing either reason or personal experience over other factors?

- What was my first day of school like? Would I have been able to ride a school bus if I had chosen to; did someone make a special trip to bring me to school? What do I remember about starting school and was my presence controversial to other families or children? Am I/was I home schooled at least in part because a public school education posed challenges with access or acceptance?

Notes

1 Self-awareness can be indicated by the ability to look in a mirror and realize one is seeing one's self, as opposed to looking in a mirror and thinking one is seeing another being. A YouTube search of kitten and puppy videos will show that dogs and cats are not self-aware; primates such as orangutans and bonobos do seem to be self-aware, for example, does one use a mirror for grooming one's self or does one react to the reflection as a potential best friend or enemy?
2 http://www.cappe.edu.au/staff/peter-singer.htm (2014); http://uchv.princeton.edu/people/faculty.php (2014).
3 *A Disability History of the United States* is a valuable resource for understanding the nuanced history of disability in the U.S. and how politics, laws, and social practices have continually fluxuated. Nielsen (2012) also shares specific examples of how the double-edged sword of prejudice against Native Americans and the disabled harmed Native disabled people, often under the guise of "educating" them.
4 http://www2.ed.gov/policy/speced/leg/idea/history.html, viewed November 11, 2013.

4
Disability Services and Higher Education

Abstract: *Disability Rights activists/students such as Ed Roberts were at the forefront of regaining access to education for people with disabilities; this growing social movement would also work to change dominant social views about accessibility. As laws changed universities found themselves dealing with students they were unprepared for while also under new legal mandates to make educational settings accessible. The Disability Services field grew from a movement begun by the first generation of university staff suddenly appointed to be service providers, when they began gathering to share best practices and ideas for how to serve the growing population of students with disabilities. Also discussed are the role of the OCR and the professionalization of the field of Disability Services, including development of a field-specific conference and journal.*

Keywords: Disability Rights and education; Disability Services and the OCR; professionalization of disability services

Oslund, Christy M. *Disability Services and Disability Studies in Higher Education: History, Contexts, and Social Impacts.* New York: Palgrave MacMillan, 2015.
DOI: 10.1057/9781137502445.0006.

Attending an institution of higher education is considered a civil right in most northern societies. Anyone who can meet entrance requirements ought to be able to get an education. What students with disabilities have traditionally found, however, was that being able to exceed the entrance requirements—looking good on paper—did not mean that universities and colleges were willing to accommodate the visibly or invisibly disabled once they arrived on campus. As Gerard Quinn (2013) observed in the Foreword he wrote for Rimmerman's *Social Inclusion of People with Disabilities*,

> It has been remarked that persons with disabilities—especially those with intellectual disabilities—are just emerging from a form of "civil death" throughout the world. Instead of being regarded as 'objects' to be managed or cared for, they are finally being acknowledged and treated as autonomous human 'subjects' in their own right (p. ix).

Those civil liberties which northern societies tend to pride themselves on offering citizens, have not in fact been equally available to people with disabilities.

Physical barriers in classrooms, dining halls, dormitories, restrooms, and parking lots while the most visible forms of exclusion are only a small part of what makes education a hostile environment for students with disabilities. For the visibly disabled there are additionally the automatic assumptions that anyone with "that disability" (insert any visible disability into the cliché) could never be successful in "that profession" (insert any field). Those with invisible disabilities find the same prejudice when requesting accommodations; "Anyone who needs (insert accommodation) can never be successful in this field."

If we reflect for a moment on the points the previous chapters have raised, we can begin to understand that these ideas and prejudices were developed over many generations and therefore will not be easily overcome. It was students with disabilities themselves who in the process of fighting for inclusion began the act of educating their societies. It was from this movement that Disabilities Studies as a field would grow. As students were beginning to organize and universities were now finding they had new students to educate, the need for service providers within higher education suddenly grew. This was the beginning of the development of the field of Disability Services.

Push back

In *No Pity*, Joseph P. Shapiro (1993) discuses some of the pioneers, students with disabilities, who fought to gain access to education at the university level. Shapiro points out that while the University of Mississippi was very publicly being integrated in 1962, no media attention surrounded a different kind of integration that was happening on the campus of Berkeley; Ed Roberts a "postpolio quadriplegic" pushed the boundaries of accommodations that the institution was willing to provide when he became a student there the same semester of 1962 (1980, pp. 41–47). In his fight to obtain access Roberts led the way for other students with disabilities, who were originally segregated in "dorm" housing which was in fact a floor of the university hospital. This group of students became politicized—in part because they were living through the civil rights movement and witnessing the difference that strong self-advocating could make—and in part because they encountered discrimination in housing, transportation, and other everyday situations. Roberts later said in a speech,

> When I was at U.C. Berkeley in the '60's, I and almost every other student on campus became involved in the Civil Rights Movement. We were fighting for the basic rights of black people. But, during my involvement in that movement, I suddenly realized something that has since been extremely important to me—that I'm part of a minority that is as segregated and devalued as any in America's history. I am part of the disabled minority.

Realizing that an individual person with disabilities was isolated and lacking in power, Roberts and other students with disabilities formed the Center for Independent Living in 1972 (Shapiro, 1993, p. 53). As he became more active Roberts began interacting with politicians; in 1975 Roberts was appointed California's director of the Department of Rehabilitation (1980, p. 54). Through his position Roberts was now able to work with disability activists from other regions of the country and he brought a young Judy Heumann, a disability activist from New York, to California to run the Center for Independent Living, where she was deputy director until 1982 (p. 58). In 1970 Heumann had sued the New York City Board of Education which had denied her teaching certificate on the basis that they did not think she would be able to get herself or her students out of a building in the case of fire [Heumann used a wheelchair], despite the fact that Heumann had successfully completed her degree and was otherwise qualified to teach (Shapiro, 1993, p. 57; Polioplace, 2011). In the out of court settlement that was reached Heumann's certification was granted. In 1983 Heumann, Roberts, and Joan Leon founded the World Institute on Disability to increase the outreach and collaboration amongst members of the disability rights and education movement (Polioplace, 2011).

Activists with disabilities working together and discovering firsthand the limits of opportunities and access available for people with disabilities—as students and citizens—would become a catalyst for further change. While not all disability activists were disabled, those with disabilities speaking and advocating on their own behalf were a large segment of the disability activist community, just as women made up the largest portion of the feminist movement. In personally experiencing prejudice and obstacles that stood in the way of access to basic opportunities such as education, people who might not otherwise have become political were pushed to take a stand for human rights, insisting that their disability not be used as an excuse to deny them their humanity.

Legalizing access

As previously mentioned, without codification in the law, access can fade out as well as in. In response to the growing social pressure for change, the U.S. federal government began to pass legislation. *The Architectural Barriers Act of 1968* mandated that buildings built, modified, or leased with federal funds were to become physically accessible for the disabled.[1] *The Rehabilitation Act of 1973* contained section 504, which included the following clause:

No otherwise qualified individual with a disability in the United States, as defined in section 705 (20) of this title, shall, solely by reason of his or her disability, be excluded from the participation in, be denied the benefits of, or be subjected to discrimination under any program or activity receiving Federal financial assistance or under any program or activity conducted by any Executive agency or by the United States Postal Service.[2]

This meant that neither public schools nor publicly funded colleges/universities could turn away a student due to the student being identified as disabled. At the higher education level, this required implementing accommodations that previously would not have been given, or that might have been available on a haphazard basis with no standard of access from one school to another, or even from one student to another within the same school. The U.S. government was beginning to follow social impetus to create universal access to education throughout the country, which would replace the regional access that was available in some areas and not in others. California had, for example, been a leader in accessibility in response to disability advocates and students with disabilities' pressure. Why should an American citizen, who happened to live with a disability and wanted to pursue a college education, for example, have to travel to California?

There was considerable conflict and question about how to meet the needs of students with disabilities. As young people who would have been prevented from obtaining an education were now fighting for access, students began to arrive at university presenting requests for services that were new to educators and administrators. In 1978 the National Council on Disability Education (NCD) was established as an advisory board to the Department of Education, as part of a revision to the Rehabilitation Act of 1973.[3] In 1984 the NCD became an independent agency responsible for reviewing "all federal disability programs and policies" expanding oversight from education alone (NCD). While there was growing legal precedence for students with disabilities to expect access to education, there was a lack of clarity amongst educational institutions about how to go about providing services. Institutions realized they needed to appoint a point person who would be responsible for implementing a standard of access across the institution; service providers realized they needed to be in dialogue in order to share best practices, discuss interpretation and application of the changing legal mandate, and to create a source of educational information for themselves.

Professional networks for disability service providers

Those professionals at the higher education level who were tapped to become the first generation of disability service providers found they were creating a field as they went. It became apparent that opportunities to share information, resources, responses, and practices would be invaluable. The Association on Higher Education and Disability® held their first annual conference in 1977 (AHEAD, 2013). What began with 100 service providers in Arizona gathering to exchange educational information and best practices grew into a national conference which would eventually attract service providers from other nations as participants and members. According to the AHEAD website, "About AHEAD":

> At this time, we boast more than 2,700 members throughout the United States, Canada, England, Australia, Ireland, Northern Ireland, New Zealand, South Africa, Sweden, Japan, and Greece. In addition to our International membership, AHEAD is fortunate to have formal partnerships with 30 Regional Affiliates and numerous other professional organizations working to advance equity in higher education for people with disabilities.

The membership of AHEAD is made up primarily of those who work at institutions of higher education and are responsible for providing accommodations and ensuring access for students with disabilities (in Chapter 1 we identified this work/role under the category of *professional staff* employed by institutions of higher education). Members of AHEAD also include legal advocates, such as Jo Anne Simon a founding member of AHEAD who was also counsel for Dr. Marilyn Bartlett in the groundbreaking case *Bartlett v. NYS Board of Law Examiners*. Also a member is Paul Grossman, for many years the Chief Regional Civil Rights Attorney for the U.S. Department of Education, Office for Civil Rights in San Francisco (AHEAD, 2012; UC Hastings, 2013). Grossman was also the founder of UC Hastings disability law program (UC Hastings, 2013). While some legal experts might have been invested in protecting institutions from the "demands" of students with disabilities, those who became involved in AHEAD were interested in assisting those with disabilities pursue social justice and access to education.

AHEAD, while the largest professional network, is not the only network that provides support for service providers in higher education. For example, there is the Australian Disability Clearing House on Education and Training (ADCET); the Canadian Association of Disability Service Providers in Post-secondary Education (CADSPPE); and for Europe the online site, the European Disability Forum (EDF), is a gathering place for advocates to share resources. What AHEAD has managed to do is create several platforms for providing support and information for service providers. AHEAD hosts a web site which stores amongst other things their code of ethics, legal decisions related to education and disability, and articles. They also sponsor an annual conference which meets in July and is hosted by different institutions/service providers/cities each year.

This conference provides continuing education opportunities and credits for service providers; annual updates on significant legal decisions; and access to learning about new technologies that facilitate the educational process for a range of students with disabilities. Smaller gatherings are also sponsored each fall and spring in the form of workshops and management institutes.

I attended my first AHEAD conference within months of being hired as a disability services specialist. I was quickly learning that my profession would require me to know something about many things: As often first contact for students and families I am both the face of the university and the intake person who receives and reviews medical documentation; it is my job to decide based on documentation and discussion with the student what "reasonable" accommodations are necessary in order to assure the student has access to campus, classrooms, and material (and I am responsible to my employer to be mindful of the difference between "reasonable" and unfeasible[4]); I am called on to negotiate between students and professors, as well as families and students, and families and the university. It was encouraging to find that in the presentations offered at my first AHEAD conference, there were information and sessions which were useful for all these applications. I was also surprised and felt better about my own preparation when I listened to fellow conference attendees explaining the backgrounds they had come from and realized that almost no one had been specially/specifically prepared for the work we were doing—we were all learning as we went and those with more experience shared with those of us who were new.

It is interesting to note that while for many years this profession drew people from other fields, we are more recently seeing an exponential growth in the final stage of "field formation"—specialized classes and degrees being offered by colleges and universities. A few examples would include: Indiana University of Pennsylvania offers a B.S. in Disability Services; Prince William Sound Community College in Alaska offers an Associate of Applied Science Degree—Disability (AAS); the University of North Florida offers a Master of Education (MEd) in Special Education, focusing on Disability Services. A range of degree types being offered in diverse geographic locations indicate that university and colleges are recognizing that disability services is not just a professional field but also a field that will continue to grow, attracting future students into the field to study.

What is a disability services specialist?

The titles disability specialists are given vary from school to school: Coordinator, Director, Assistant Dean of Students being some of the more common. The office title also varies although wording often includes Disability Services and Academic Support Services. The responsibilities of a disability support specialist include but are not limited to:

- Meeting with students and reviewing their documentation of disability.
- Determining in collaboration with the individual student what supports will be appropriate for academic success/access.
- Ensuring that the necessary services and supports are provided.
- Monitoring physical accessibility of the campus including residence halls and dining rooms.
- Providing technology/resources that bridge gaps in information delivery (closed captioning, etc.).

Some schools have well-staffed offices that can provide sign language interpreters, note takers, alternate book formats, technical support, and academic support councilors. Most offices, however, are not large and may need to contract with outside service providers for some services. Not all schools have the resources to offer the same services.

The disability services specialist works with a range of people across campus and the community. For example, I will work regularly with faculty and students negotiating alternate assignments and test accommodations. I provide education and training for faculty and staff related to diversity, disability, and universal design. I work with students on academic skill building including time management and study skills. Every week I spend time talking to parents who are concerned about how best to support their students; I also answer numerous questions from families/friends who have students still in the K-12 system regarding how to prepare students for college. Like all administrators, I also spend time in meetings and on committees supporting the mission and goals of the institution. There are also regular legal changes, decisions, and rulings from the Office of Civil Rights (OCR) related to disability services that a specialist needs to keep abreast of, as each of these cases further clarifies expectations that the government has of institutions. Other members of the campus community will often look to the disability services specialist on their campus for advice on when classroom or campus practices could potentially be infringing on students' rights, or conversely, to clarify just how much they must to do to meet students' requests.

The Office of Civil Rights (OCR)[5]

The OCR responds to complaints filed by people who feel a school/program has treated them in a discriminatory manner and not rectified the discrimination when it was brought to the institution's administrative attention. Complaints can cover almost anything: Being dismissed from a program of study; being treated differently than other students; not being given a required accommodation; not being allowed a service or therapy animal or having restricted access to spaces when in the company of said animal; being required to use technology that isn't accessible, etc.

The OCR's primary focus is ensuring access. When an institution's programs, spaces, or policies are discriminatory then the OCR focus is on making the needed alterations to ensure access is improved. This may mean a university revises a policy, revisits a decision, more clearly explicates a process/policy, or remodels a space. Often the OCR works with an institution to ensure changes that are improvements to accessibility. While there have been cases where students have received considerations that have a monetary value, this is usually in the form of being allowed to repeat classes without paying additional tuition. The OCR generally does not require schools to give students money—they work toward providing the student access and often students find that what they feel has been a discriminatory action falls within acceptable policy ranges and is not a violation of law. Being disabled and dissatisfied with how one has been treated does not equate to being discriminated against. Institutions have more power than individual students; the OCR's role is to assist students when institutions are not responding to necessary access to education. Unfortunately for those of us with disabilities, the OCR continues to be vitally necessary as there remains a bias in place which favors those who are not disabled. If things have "always been done this way" for persons without disabilities, people can be reluctant or unable to see why revisions are necessary to make a process more accessible.

Disability service providers are ideally meant to have roles that *are not* limited to ensuring student accommodations. They should also be given opportunities to educate their campus about increasing accessibility. From a practical point of view though, some offices have so few resources in both human-hours and financial support that they are already stretched too thin. *Educating the campus* is one area where collaboration with disability studies could prove beneficial to all parties.

Disability services specialists also will spend time educating students and families about the changing nature of services when a student begins college-level study. It is natural that a family and student's expectations will be informed by what they experienced in the kindergarten to grade 12 (K-12) system. The mandate of including all students in education, which the K-12 schools are responsible for however, differs from that of university. College-level education is designed to be accessible for "qualified students" and does not require professors to fundamentally alter expectations within the class.[6] In application this means that accommodations which might have been commonplace in primary or secondary school will suddenly no longer be available to a student once they are in college. One example of this would be the use of calculators in math classes.

It is not uncommon for students with dysgraphia, dyslexia, and other processing disorders to use calculators for all math-related work in secondary school. These students and their families expect this accommodation to carry over into college-level work. Part of the disability specialist's job is to explain the circumstances where this is not possible, even though use of a calculator may otherwise be part of a student's accommodations. One of the Calculus classes on the campus where I work, for example, has two sections to the exams they give during the course of the semester: one section of the exam is designed to test a student's ability to work an equation without a calculator. No student is allowed to use a calculator on the noncalculator section of the exam—even if otherwise the calculator is allowed as an accommodation. In this particular class the use of calculators is restricted when the ability to process functions is what the student is being tested on. In other words, students *are being tested* on their ability to process symbols. When one has a processing disorder this can appear to be a discriminatory test. This class is part of a series of classes though, that is preparing students to become a professional in science or engineering where the ability to process symbols may exclude people with particular types of disabilities from being successful in the field. Would the OCR find this class to be discriminatory and require the professor or university to alter the class?

It is unlikely. Some expectations are considered in keeping with the type of knowledge that a student would be expected to have when working within their respective field.[7] A surgeon, for example, is expected to have the parts of a human body memorized and a professional mathematician is expected to have certain formulas memorized.

If on the other hand, a professor in the English department were to place a math question on their exam and not allow a student with an accommodation for calculators to use a calculator because "no one gets to use a calculator" the student would have a reason for talking to first their professor, then their disability services specialist if necessary. The teaching goals of an English class and instructor are different than in math; each field of study has accepted standards of practice, and while the teaching goals may sometimes overlap (all instructors like to encourage "good writing" from students, even if they disagree about what "good writing" is) some practices would be considered outside a field's established standard practices.

The work of the disability services specialist may at times include stepping in when a student is not being treated equitably and assist in resolving issues. This work sometimes requires a specialist to sit down with a professor to discuss the goal, or pedagogical purpose of an assignment, and then work with the professor and student to find possible ways to meet that goal in a nondiscriminatory fashion. I can think of an example from my own work: A professor in a chemistry class was requiring students to write out journal entries. On the surface, the assignment in and of itself was not discriminatory; however, one of the students in the class was dyslexic and he was finding the assignment very difficult and time consuming. When he approached the professor and explained this she said she was willing to work with the student; however, she was not sure how to proceed or alter the assignment. After all, she explained, she was expecting all students to do the same work, so didn't that make the assignment "fair"?

The student, professor, and I sat down together. I talked to the professor about her pedagogical purpose for the assignment—what was she expecting everyone in the class to learn or demonstrate they were learning by giving them this assignment? Once we had clarified the kind of knowledge the students were expected to be demonstrating (analysis of lab results), the three of us together were able to brainstorm other ways for the student with dyslexia to show he was capable of doing this work. Ideally, this is the type of conflict resolution that a student, professor, and university take part in, rather than having things reach the level of requiring OCR intervention. Disability service providers ought to work in a climate of supportive practices. When necessary there should be conversations regarding the difference between pedagogical practices which support the work and practices within a field, and practices which are still being used simply because "that's how we've always done it."

One of the tools that can be helpful in a disability services specialist's work is membership in a professional organization like AHEAD and keeping updated on best practices within the field. This assists a service provider not only because he or she then has access to a number of resources but because one will also learn the importance of clarifying the mission and purpose of their own office in relation to the work of the institution they work for and with. Being a member of a profession with a code of ethics can provide guidance should an individual feel conflicted between their employer's goals and the goals of the work they have been employed to carry out.

Ethics, Professional, and Program Standards

AHEAD has worked over the years to develop a Code of Ethics, a set of Professional Standards, and Program Standards which a service provider and disability services office may use as guidelines. Having such standards are not only part of developing a professional field, they also allow service providers to measure their own programs and services compared to expectations within the field. As Thomas Kuhn observed when explaining his theory of how paradigm shifts occur within a field, it is the consensus of the field that decides which practices are valid, which are mainstream, and which are outside accepted practices (Kuhn, 1962). One must be a participant within the field to fully understand the field's expectations, goals, and accepted standards. New members to a field become participants within the field in part by learning and internalizing the field's standards and taking part in the practices that the field endorses.

As one becomes familiar with the disability services field, one will find that the focus is on supporting inclusive practices and standards, which will facilitate, "the highest levels of educational excellence and potential quality of life for postsecondary students with disabilities" (AHEAD, Code). *The Standards and Performance Indicators* provide a point by point explanation of the purpose and goals of a "Service Disability Specialist"; included here is the outline of these standards (detailed PDF with examples available at http://www.ahead.org/learn/resources):

1. Consultation/Collaboration
   1.1 Serve as an advocate for issues regarding students with disabilities to ensure equal access.
   1.2 Provide disability representation on relevant campus committees.
2. Information Dissemination
   2.1 Disseminate information through institutional electronic and printed publications regarding disability services and how to access them.
   2.2 Provide services that promote access to the campus community.
   2.3 Disseminate information to students with disabilities regarding available campus and community disability resources.
3. Faculty Staff Awareness
   3.1 Inform faculty regarding academic accommodations, compliance with legal responsibilities as well as instructional, programmatic, and curriculum modifications.
   3.2 Provide consultation with administrators regarding academic accommodations, compliance with legal responsibilities, as well as instructional, programmatic, physical, and curriculum modifications.
   3.3 Provide disability awareness training for campus constituencies such as faculty, staff, and administrators.
   3.4 Provide information to faculty about services available to students with disabilities.
4. Academic Adjustments
   4.1 Maintain records that document the student's plan for the provision of selected accommodations.
   4.2 Determine with students appropriate academic accommodations and services.
   4.3 Collaborate with faculty to ensure that reasonable academic accommodations do not fundamentally alter the program of study.
5. Counseling and Self-Determination
   5.1 Use a service delivery model that encourages students with disabilities to develop independence.

6. Policies and Procedures
   6.1 Develop, review, and revise written policies and guidelines regarding procedures for determining and accessing "reasonable accommodations."
   6.2 Assist with the development, review, and revision of written policies and guidelines for institutional rights and responsibilities with respect to service provision.
   6.3 Develop, review, and revise written policies and guidelines for student rights and responsibilities with respect to receiving services.
   6.4 Develop, review, and revise written policies and guidelines regarding confidentiality of disability information.
   6.5 Assist with the development, review, and revision of policies and guidelines for settling a formal complaint regarding the determination of a "reasonable accommodation."
7. Program Administration and Evaluation
   7.1 Provide services that are aligned with the institution's mission or services philosophy.
   7.2 Coordinate services for students with disabilities through a full-time professional.
   7.3 Collect student feedback to measure satisfaction with disability services.
   7.4 Collect data to monitor use of disability services.
   7.5 Report program evaluation data to administrators.
   7.6 Provide fiscal management of the office that serves students with disabilities.
   7.7 Collaborate in establishing procedures for purchasing the adaptive equipment needed to assure equal access.
8. Training and Professional Development
   8.1 Provide disability services staff with ongoing opportunities for professional development.
   8.2 Provide services by personnel with training and experience working with college students with disabilities (e.g., student development, degree programs).
   8.3 Assure that personnel adhere to relevant Codes of Ethics (e.g., AHEAD, APA).

These standards have evolved with the field and reflect the "maturation" of the profession.

People with disabilities within the field

As a person with disabilities/disabled person I do occasionally sit in conference rooms and feel like people are speaking *about* those of us who are disabled as opposed to speaking with us, or as speaking from a position of lived experience. This of course is not always true, and is less true in AHEAD meetings than when I first joined. This does, however, lead to two points. First, while there have always been some individuals with disabilities within the field of disability services, many of those who work in the field would not consider themselves disabled. Best intentions aside, it is worth considering what it means to a field when it primarily developed with those identified as nondisabled "serving" people identified as disabled. How might this impact interactions between service providers and students, students who are already in a less powerful position, and who also are identified as disabled must *ask* professional staff to facilitate their access to education?

Second, it is worth mentioning that the interests of the institutions that disability services specialists are employed by may at times be in conflict with the interests of individual students with disabilities. Students want an education; while some students are interested in education as a matter of quality of life, most are pursuing education with the idea of obtaining a degree and a career. Individuals want the opportunity to try any field they are interested in or passionate about; institutions want to manage processes and expectations so that students complete a program of study within a limited time frame. Some institutions will have concerns about "cost effectiveness," and with "time to completion rates" meaning they want the numbers to reflect that most students finish a degree [undergraduate] in four to five years, and bring in tuition money without costing more-than-average in services used. Students with disabilities may find themselves under pressure from the institution to switch their course of study, leave with certification as opposed to a baccalaureate degree, or transfer to a "less challenging" institution or program of study. Service specialists may at times find themselves mediators in negotiations between their employers and their clients; ethically the student comes first and practically this can make relations with an employer uncomfortable.

To illustrate how students with disabilities sometimes do not fit within "normal" university expectations I will use an example from my own academic background. When I was working on my doctoral degree my language processing disability complicated my dissertation completion. Departments typically make funding available to doctoral students, often in return for the doctoral student either teaching classes or carrying out research. There is also typically a limit to how many years funding is available to an individual, because departments need to be able to recruit new graduate students. I used most of the funding available to me through my department and ended up going to work full time while completing my degree, in order to keep my education/life funded. I also finished my degree in the final semester I had available to do so before it would have been *mandated* by the institution's graduate school that I write for permission to extend beyond the allowed "time to degree completion." In other words, students have a limited number of years they are allowed (eight years in my program) to complete their degree; it is considered another "sign" that one might not be suitable for their intended field of study if they cannot complete their degree in the allotted time. If I had exceeded my timeline and had needed to write a request for an extension, then it would have been possible that my request would have been denied. It was more than theoretically possible that I would have put seven years of class work, research, and writing into a degree without receiving one. A disability specialist could have helped me negotiate an extension to my timeline, in part through education of the institution's policy makers regarding the impact the disability I live with has on my writing process.

Chapter 4: Thought points

- At certain historical points students were expected to memorize everything that was told to them and then be able to verbally repeat what they had heard (without the aid of any writing); think about all the ways that current students aid their memory of material. Would I as a student be at a disadvantage/advantage if I were suddenly expected to memorize all material without any support besides hearing the teacher speak? What assists me in being the most effective learner I can be? What educational practices frustrate my attempts to learn?
- How would students and the classroom environment be affected if only half of students in each class were given access to textbooks,

notes, and desks? What would the different impacts be on the two groups of students both those who had access while their peers did not and those who were denied access? Can I observe limits in access in my current educational context or in an educational context I am aware of?

▸ The OCR is specific to the U.S.; identify legal resources students in other nations could appeal to if they were being discriminated against in trying to access an education. What supports are specific to the nation in which I live?

▸ What accommodations do the college I attend or work at, or that is in/nearest to my community offer for students? What can I learn about these services by visiting the institution's web site? After accessing the web site do I have a clear understanding of how to obtain accommodations?

Notes

1 PL 90–480.
2 PL 93–112.
3 The Rehabilitation Act is part of the Labor Code; referenced as U.S.C., Title 29.
4 "Unfeasible" can be related to issues caused by our geographic isolation and northern climate. It is reasonable to replace a heavy door with an automatic electronic door to improve an access point, but not to provide a personal attendant to shovel the snow for each individual as they attempt to cross campus during a regular winter storm.
5 The OCR is specific to the U.S. and has influenced the development of the disability services field through legal rulings and investigative powers. Many nations and the UN have also passed laws which protect the rights of access for people with disabilities, an area also known as Human Rights Law. Syracuse University provides resources regarding other nation-state's laws related to disability: http://www.law.syr.edu/library/electronic-resources/legal-research-guides/humanrights.aspx
6 What makes a student qualified to be present is increasingly murky: Students who are very intelligent but struggle with social conduct, or with fulfilling the range of general education classes outside their area of interest are examples of students who push the notion of what qualifies a student for academic presence. How we approach higher education, including preparing people for careers, seems to require further redesign.

7 Students in this situation argue that in "the real world" they will always have access to calculators and calculating applications on computers and that therefore this is an archaic method of testing people. Are math tests that rely on paper/pencil one day going to go the way that dexterity with the abacus has gone, with only a few practitioners in the future fluent with such methods?

5
Disability Studies and Higher Education

Abstract: *Beginning with the Union of Physically Impaired Against Segregation, foundational documents were produced which stated for larger social consumption the concerns as voiced by people with disabilities. As those with disabilities fought to speak on their own behalf, their concerns were naturally brought into classrooms where they were teaching and also raised by allies in teaching contexts. Professionalization of the field included development of groups such as the Society for Disability Studies, conferences, and a journal.*

Keywords: people with disabilities speak/write; professionalization of disability studies; Union of Physically Impaired Against Segregation

Oslund, Christy M. *Disability Services and Disability Studies in Higher Education: History, Contexts, and Social Impacts.* New York: Palgrave MacMillan, 2015.
DOI: 10.1057/9781137502445.0007.

Disability Studies refers generally to the examination of disability as a social, cultural, and political phenomenon. In contrast to clinical, medical, or therapeutic perspectives on disability, Disability Studies focuses on how disability is defined and represented in society. It rejects the perception of disability as a functional impairment that limits a person's activities. From this perspective, disability is not a characteristic that exists in the person or a problem of the person that must be "fixed" or "cured." Instead, disability is a construct that finds its meaning within a social and cultural context.

The Center on Human Policy, Law, and Disability Studies Syracuse University

There are different pieces to the origin of the development of disability studies as an academic area of study, reflective in part of the fact that disability studies grew differently in each nation. A commonality which has been shown in the previous chapters is that people with disabilities had been dislocated from public places, institutionalized, and stripped of human rights. Disability activists and students with disabilities had fought to obtain access to what was named but was not in fact *public education* for young children. They then had to fight for access to college education, a fight which started in earnest during the 1960s; the fight to make education more accessible continues to this day. A significant role has also been played by *written documents* which served as iconic statements by people with disabilities. These documents began to clarify for the larger society why people with disabilities were rejecting the traditional role that society had tried to force them into, a role where they required care and services without a voice in their own futures or fates. Documents also allowed those with disabilities to clarify shared interests, providing focus and rallying points which could be used to inform changes to legislation and social practices.

Important early writings

Two foundational documents originated in the UK with the Union of the Physically Impaired Against Segregation (UPIAS). In 1974 UPIAS members wrote and published their Foundation Statement, which can now be found online at the Center for Disability Studies, University of Leeds,[1] and at libcom.org.[2] Adopted in 1974 and amended in 1976 this Statement both gave voice to concerns of people with disabilities, while also clarifying for the larger public what was identified as the disabling social construct that society was placing them in. The Statement also identified the disabled people that UPIAS identified as their primary membership: Full membership being open to those with "*physical impairment* [emphasis added]... This is because we believe the important thing at the moment is to clarify the facts of our situation and the problems associated with physical impairment" (point 22). While others could join as associate members, only full members were allowed to vote on Union business.

The Union also pledged (point 27) to work with and also in effect, hold accountable, other organizations which claimed to speak on "behalf of disabled people." It was in this role that the Union found themselves in a conversation which led to the publication of their next foundational document, *Fundamental Principles of Disability* (1975). The Union wanted clarification from The Disability Alliance, regarding the basis on which the Alliance was identifying themselves as spokespeople for the disabled. The Alliance claimed to be an "umbrella organization" representing groups that spoke on *behalf of* people with disabilities. As Vic Finkelstein, a representative of UPIAS, asked pointedly of the Alliance representatives during their meeting, "What have you done to actually involve disabled people" (*Fundamental*, p. 8). One of the primary spokesmen for the Alliance (represented at the meeting by four able-bodied men) Peter Townsend replied that "We are publishing material of concern to disabled people" (p. 8).

The summary of the meeting along with select quotes, followed by commentary from both groups was printed and distributed. The commentary from UPIAS makes clear that it is time for people with disabilities to be heard, without the "experts" such as Alliance members deciding what social and policy priorities ought to be for those with disabilities. While the members of the Alliance were interested in identifying degrees of disability within individuals as a basis for deciding how much aid an individual should be eligible for, the members of UPIAS, that is, the people who were themselves disabled, wanted to switch the focus from individual impairment to the social construct of disability which discriminated against all people identified as disabled. This discussion and these documents were foundational in the development of the social justice model of disability.

In the U.S., a significant document was then commissioned by the World Rehabilitation Fund, Inc. and written by Vic Finkelstein. *Attitudes and Disabled People* addressed social issues that Finkelstein pointed out were ubiquitous to the context of disability. Published in 1980 the monograph was part of a series of monographs designed to respond to the passage of the Rehabilitation Act of 1973 (Finkelstein, 1980, Preface). By this point Finkelstein had further refined the theme which would become core to disability studies and which he captures in the document Summary.

The central thesis of this monograph is that "disability" is an oppressive social relationship. Its focus is attitudes toward "disability." Prevalent attitudes, however, are only uncovered as a result of research or social analysis. It is argued that those who carry out research or social analysis of necessity participate in the "disabling social relationship." What we know about attitudes, therefore, cannot be separated from the conditions in which they are uncovered. The monograph aims to encourage service deliverers to adopt a more critical attitude toward their own participation in the disability relationship. It also seeks to encourage a more critical attitude toward views which treat the subject matter in isolation from the definite historical social relationship in which such attitudes are uncovered. While the social model remains the dominate model in disability studies, not everyone has the same definition of what exactly the social model represents; there is however, some core common agreement, that is, one cannot consider what "disability" means outside of the social context where the label of disability is being applied. There is also some disagreement over where the future focus of the field should be, a point we will return to shortly.

Dissention/discussion

Vic Finkelstein and Mike Oliver are generally considered two of the more prominent (though certainly not the only) writers in the development of disability studies in the UK; both authors have also proven internationally influential (Ferguson and Nusbaum, 2012; Shakespeare, 2013). Finkelstein played a key role in UPIAS documents, while Oliver is credited with originating the term "social model" and is a tireless advocate of a strong social model. Oliver wrote in 2013, "Critics of the social model began to emerge soon after I coined the term" and while the original criticism was from the experts who wanted to continue to define what disability and related concerns were, the criticism eventually started to come from some "disabled people and academics working in disability studies."[3] One of the critics that Oliver is referencing would doubtless have to be Tom Shakespeare.

Shakespeare posits that in the U.S., Canada, Australia, "and other countries" the theory of the social model has a "looser social-contextual concept" with a "minority group approach" while he identifies the British version as a "strong social model" (2013, p. 11). Shakespeare points to the statement by UPIAS which said:

> In our view, it is society which disables physically impaired people. Disability is something imposed on top of our impairments, by the way we are unnecessarily isolated and excluded from full participation in society. (2013, p. 12)

Shakespeare agrees that historically this strong social model was "crucial" to the disability movement.[4] He also argues that the strong social model needs to adjust [or redesign] in order to remain relevant to current concerns in the disability movement and to the lives of people with disabilities.

Shakespeare's predominate criticisms of a strong social model are:

▸ It tends to force all disabled people [UPIAS/UK preferred terminology] into one homogeneous group; all are oppressed "regardless of impairment" (Shakespeare, 2013, p. 17).
▸ "The role of rehabilitation is summarily dismissed" because rehabilitation focuses on the individual and the proper focus should be on social change (Shakespeare, 2013, p. 18).
▸ Rather than meeting the needs of individuals the focus becomes removing social barriers; the importance of individual experience is decreased as is the realization of either the number of people with specific disabilities or how their needs should impact funding priorities (Shakespeare, 2013, p. 19).

Oliver, on the other hand, counters that it is precisely the focus on individual impairment which the social model was meant to avoid, "Our differences are being used to slash our services" he argues, and places the blame on a weakening of the social model (*Disability Now*). In Oliver's words, "Disabled people urgently need a reinvigorated social model—or something new to replace it." Oliver makes it clear that to "talk down" the social model without leaving something substantial and even better in its place once again leads to discrimination against people with disabilities.

Shakespeare also bemoans the current UK government's choice to cut benefits and yet points out that "the differences between disabled people are as important as the similarities" (2013, p. 239). Shakespeare prods for "engaged social research" which provides evidence for how "disabled people experience barriers" (ibid.). While he has criticisms of the strong social model Shakespeare also clearly outlines his agreement with the current shared understandings:

- That social and environmental barriers constitute major problems.
- Disabled people should have choices and be supported to live in the community.
- Medicalization/assumptions limiting disabled people must be challenged (2013, p. 238).

Ongoing discussions and disagreements within the disabilities studies/disability movement should therefore not be seen as emanating from vastly different understandings of some of the key concerns experienced by people with disabilities. Rather, the disagreements tend to be more subtle: Should political focus include discussion of "individual impairment" or should a broader focus be maintained which emphasizes the social context that all which is labeled disabled entails; do "experts" have a role in the discussion and what does it mean to be an expert; what is the disability rights movement to gain/lose if groups identify by disability rather than speaking with a more unified voice on behalf of all who are labeled disabled? These are questions which will continue to be debated.

Professional networks

The Society for Disability Studies is an academic/scholarly organization which has international membership; however, their physical headquarters are in North Carolina (in Chapter 1 we identified these people as primarily *faculty*, responsible for education; this includes those who develop and deliver classroom content). According to the organization's web site, they trace their origin to 1982 and their initial incarnation as the Section for the Study of Chronic Illness, Impairment, and Disability (SSCIID);[5] they took their current name in 1986 (Society). Disability Studies is an interdisciplinary field and as such both classes offered in the field and degrees available in the field vary across institutions. As of this writing, nearly 40 U.S. and Canadian universities were offering degrees related to disability studies. Syracuse University keeps an updated web site which lists current U.S./Canadian programs: http://disabilitystudies.syr.edu/resources/programsinds.aspx.

Obviously when a field is made up of practitioners who actually come from a range of backgrounds, there may be some variation in how they would describe the field. As Ferguson and Nusbaum (2012) point out in "Disability Studies: What is it and What Difference Does it Make" it might be easier to say what Disability Studies is not. They do, however, identify five hallmarks of the kind of work that belongs in the Disability Studies field [or a disabilities studies program]:

- It must be social.
- It must be foundational, that is, fundamental to our understanding of ourselves and how we identify difference and sameness.
- It must be interdisciplinary.
- It must be participatory, for example, people with disabilities are participants.
- It must be values-based, considering the ethical implications of what is done (pp. 72–75).

It is also important to note that while it is typical for a disability studies program to be built on a social model, as previously pointed out, the social model is open to different interpretations based on the nation, institution, and other lenses that focus a discussion.

While the Society for Disability Studies is an international, multidisciplinary organization, it is not the only organization for people within the disability studies field. Further examples of associations include The Canadian Disabilities Studies Association; the Disability Studies and Research Institute, Sydney, Australia; and Disability Rights UK. The Center for Disability Studies at Leeds University, founded by professor and activist Colin Barnes, also provides an important online archive of articles and material related to the disability rights movement (http://disability-studies.leeds.ac.uk/).

How does one enter the field?

Arguably, the pioneers of the disabilities studies field did not set out to found a field of study; they were speaking about their own experiences, and attempting to educate the public about the social exclusion they were experiencing on a daily basis. It was natural for those who were part of this movement and also educators to bring these discussions into the classroom. At the same time, some educators did begin to develop classes which tried to change the lens through which students looked at social experiences, attempting to raise awareness of the differences between what we consider "normal" and what we label "disabled" and how these concepts tie into identity, portrayals in popular media, design, accessibility, basically any and all areas of life. If we reflect on what we have previously seen regarding religion, philosophy, politics, law, and popular culture having all influenced the northern social view regarding stigmatization and disability, it should be clearer at this point why the work of disability studies had become so necessary. There were thousands of years of social practices and beliefs founded on bias that had led to a need for educating people about social views they took for granted.

As a result, classes that can count for credit toward a degree in Disability Studies can cover a range of topics, and people are graduating with a variety of specializations. Perhaps equally importantly, students who are not specializing in the field now have an increasing possibility of encountering course content which includes information generated by the Disability Studies field, as the field grows and develops.

Education cannot be truly *diverse* if students are not having opportunities to engage in conversations and learning about what it means to be disabled in their society. There was once a time, for example, when someone would be considered well educated if they knew only about the writings and accomplishments of a list of white males. As we continue to recognize all the contributions and stories such a view of history ignores, we realize that another part of what has been missing in our traditional telling of history is the influence that people we would identify as disabled have had. In turn, recognizing that people who lived with disability were accomplishing significant things (or living ordinary lives like others) challenges our current views of what it means to be "disabled."

Fields within Disability Studies

Given the interdisciplinary nature of the larger disability studies field, it seems fitting that many of the degrees offered are also interdisciplinary. Some of the areas of focus include: Arts, Humanities, Education, and Human/Family Development. Given this interdisciplinary breadth of study-possibilities, scholars can often choose a focus which suits their own interests and background, bringing a nearly endless range of possibilities to what one may study from a Disability Studies perspective.

A statement on the Disability Studies department homepage for the University of Washington provides a somewhat typical example of how universities are approaching the field and providing the range of programs necessary for a degree within the field:

> The Disability Studies Major investigates, enhances, and complements the understanding of disability by incorporating social, cultural, historical, political, legal and educational perspectives. While the conceptualization of disability changes over time, disability itself is a constant component of human existence. The Disability Studies Major was designed to provide a comprehensive curriculum in Disability Studies that includes the incorporation of the lived experiences of disabled people. (2014, University of Washington)

Canada's Ryerson University is an example of a school that makes a slightly clearer connection in their homepage statement between their social-justice framing for disability studies and active participation in the current disability rights movement. Ryerson clearly identifies the disability rights movement as foundational to their understanding of what it means to be "active" in the field.

> As scholars in Disability Studies, we consider it important to remain connected to the disability rights movement. Maintaining the "fusion" between disability studies and people with disabilities and their organizations is an important underpinning of Ryerson's Disability Studies program. (2014, Ryerson University)

Ryerson is one example of a school which identifies continuing activity within the disability rights movement as part and parcel of being an academic. At the same time, such a statement seems to beg the question—if one is studying "their organizations" than is one not finding that people with disabilities are themselves some of the key members of the faculty and student body? This is not to suggest that Ryerson lacks scholars with disabilities but rather, leads us to the next tension that is an undercurrent in the field.

As has already been alluded to, there are at times a delicate tension between those who identify as disabled and those who do not identify as a person with a disability but who do study disability. Perhaps this is exactly as it should be? Whenever we as academics, professionals, administrators, or teachers speak we speak from a position of authority.

We should be mindful of the reality that no matter how carefully we choose our words, or what our personal identity, we can never speak on behalf of everyone. There is no perfectly correct language or all inclusive concept; there are general agreements, often with slight contention over details. Perhaps our responsibility should always be to remain mindful of the limits of our individual experience and education, while doing our best to facilitate learning and discussion which further encourages people to rethink their own understanding of disability. This takes us back to a point made in the Preface: All original designs require redesign to remain viable and redesign remains a continuing process. When a way of doing, a field, a design becomes stagnant, that indicates the movement is basically "dead" and historical. That which is alive will continue to adapt. The Disability Studies field is very much alive and thus continues to undergo adaptation.

Nonetheless, there is a current of resentment among some who are disabled; concerns exist about what happens when those who do not identify as disabled, study disability and teach disability classes. Snyder and Mitchell summarize one of the primary concerns in *Cultural Locations of Disability*,

> Can disability studies and the study of disability pursue work without further contributing to the oppression of those bodies that researchers seek to know and assess—even liberate? What lessons must we take from a history of "people-based research practices" performed in the name of disabled people's best interests? (p. 195)

As with any group, there will be questions about what group membership entails and who within a group has a right to speak. Consider, for example, that the original UPIAS group only allowed full membership to those with physical disability; while others could hold supportive roles they were not allowed to vote (and thus speak) on behalf of the group. This not only excluded the nondisabled from speaking, it also excluded those whose impairment was unseen—the mentally ill, the learning disabled, etc. Those who are disabled have already fought long and hard to have their own voices heard. Those with unseen disabilities also struggle to be heard as a significant segment of the broader range of people with disabilities.

Indeed, there are some tensions between the physically disabled and those with unseen disabilities. As one of my colleagues who lives with a largely unseen disability has complained to me, "They [visibly disabled] act like we don't exist! It's bad enough society marginalizes me but when other disabled people do, just because they can't see—it really pisses me off." The more active she has become in the disability studies field and the disability rights movement, the more she has felt like a second-class citizen *also* within the disabled community.

Government and private hiring initiatives in Canada and the U.S. which have focused on increasing the number of people with disabilities in the workplace have also tended to focus on the visibly disabled, although when one of my colleagues from our Career Services Office asked a government employee about this (we had been sent literature which completely focused on accommodating the physically disabled and encouraging *their* job applications) the government representative was quick to say that anyone with a "documented" disability was welcome to apply for government work. There is a subtle code at work here: In the U.S. we are not allowed to request documentation "proving" a disability from someone who is visibly [physically] disabled; however, we are allowed to request documentation from "a certified professional" regarding those of us who live with unseen disabilities.[6] What those of us living with unseen disabilities thus can "hear"—whether it is the message intended or not—is that we cannot be given the same rights and access as the physically disabled; after all, we might be lying about our disability. Both the government and society maintain that there are "privileges" to an identity of disability that others will try to claim if the label of disability is not safeguarded. I have yet to encounter people living with disabilities on the other hand, who are being overwhelmed by the "rights and privileges" that their disability is supposed to entail. This is just another way of labeling and controlling an identity that remains stigmatized in larger social circles. Northern society continues to consider disability a problem located within individuals and insists on controlling which individuals "merit" the label of disabled.

A final point about tensions within the larger "community" of disability; historically white males have held power and been the individuals who have had a voice and platform to speak from. This is true not just in larger northern society but also within the disability rights movement. When we look at both UPIAS' writings and student activists who rose to positions of prominence during the disability rights movement from the 1960s onward, we can see that white males have dominated the movement. We can ask, why have more woman or people of color not been prominent; this is a bit like asking why more women and non-Athenians were not speaking up in the Greek assembly in ancient Athens—in order to have a voice one first must be in the room.

The inequalities that are persistent in larger society—a lack of gender equity, including equal pay for equal work, for example, are magnified within the disability rights movement. Northern academic institutions, which for so long have been dominated by white males, continue to be unbalanced regarding whose voices are given prominent platforms to speak from, in part because there remains fewer voices in the room able to speak from other perspectives. There are still very few women with disabilities and people of color with disabilities present in higher education, never mind women of color who are disabled—therefore their voices are fewer and must be more closely listened for if one is to hear from their points of view. Alison Kafer speaks to this when she talks about the importance of forming coalitions between those who remain marginalized or on the fringes. Kafer suggests that coalitions where we work "alongside each other" have potential to bring more strength to these otherwise quiet voices, which alone are easier to ignore; she is in agreement with Bearnice Johnson Reagon that "forming coalitions across differences is both necessary and terrifying" (1983/2000, p. 151). To be in a successful coalition means giving time and energy to other people's concerns, to value other people's points of view, and to act for interests that may not always align with our own. I would suggest that in a coalition we also will be forced to face any privilege we may enjoy, even as we also are in other ways marginalized.

Chapter 5: Thought points

- What area do I consider my "specialization" or the field where my knowledge is centered? What are some of the ways that disability studies and my field intersect? What classes unique to my field are available which currently consider the intersection of the field and disability? What classes do I think there ought to be?
- Can I identify a reading, display, presentation, or planned event related to disability that has had a strong impact on me? What made it memorable? What are my takeaways, or lasting ideas/impressions?
- When I am a student in a class do I think of myself as part of a learning community (why or why not)? If a classroom, discussion group, or seminar is a learning community what are my personal

responsibilities to other members of the community? How do I as an individual either contribute to other's learning or frustrate their learning?

- Kafer suggests coalitions that could include transgender people and people with disabilities, both groups who are currently marginalized in society, including academia. If you were forming a coalition within the disability rights movement, what groups/identities would you wish to have present within your coalition and why? What are several social change goals that members of this coalition might agree on?

Notes

1. "Policy Statement" (1974). http://disability-studies.leeds.ac.uk/files/library/UPIAS-UPIAS.pdf
2. "Constitution of the Union of the Physically Impaired Against Segregation", https://libcom.org/library/constitution-union-physically-impaired-against-segregation
3. (2013). "The Social Model: A Victim of Criticism." *Disability Now.* http://www.disabilitynow.org.uk/article/social-model-victim-criticism
4. Chapter 2, "Materialist Approaches to Disability" in *Disability Rights and Wrong Revisited* sets out in detail what Shakespeare identifies as two crucial pieces that developed as a result of the social movement.
5. The "section" was a group formed at a gathering of the Western Social Science Association by Darryl Evans, Gary Kiger, Stephen Hey, and John Seidel (Ferguson and Nusbaum, 2012).
6. Unless the individual is applying for a "scheduled A" government job, a process reserved for people with disabilities; the schedule A application process begins with sending in a resume, and a letter from someone qualified to state that the individual applying is disabled.

6
Barriers to Interactions between Disability Studies and Disability Services

Abstract: *This chapter explores the difference in employer expectations for faculty [professionals in Disability Studies] and staff [professionals in Disability Services] and some of the ways this impacts efforts to share collaborative projects between the fields. With limited resources of time, funding, and professional development restraints, there are some specific challenges that stand between collaborative efforts between the two fields. Is the separation of fields making a difference that matters?*

Keywords: crossing academic divides; professional resource allocation; professionally valued work

Oslund, Christy M. *Disability Services and Disability Studies in Higher Education: History, Contexts, and Social Impacts.* New York: Palgrave MacMillan, 2015. DOI: 10.1057/9781137502445.0008.

Given the separate nature of life for faculty and staff on campus which we have now established, along with the different origins and purposes of the fields of disability studies and disability services, it should by this point be no surprise that these two fields have had little overlap. Not only do the two fields have different origins, they also fulfill different roles in academia. More recently, however, individuals within both fields are deliberately fostering interdisciplinary discussions looking at ways for these previously separate areas to begin a dialogue. In this chapter we consider some of the difficulties inherent within academia that will complicate deliberate interaction between the fields. Once we have considered the difficulties, we will move on to consider why these deliberate interaction—or coalition forming—is nonetheless desirable and worth the challenges such work faces.

Work with professional value

Expectations of faculty, expectations of staff

Disability studies is an interdisciplinary field and there is already a great deal of collaborative work being done within the field. Participants, however, typically have one thing in common; they tend to be faculty. As was previously pointed out, faculty are encouraged to conduct research and publish. Faculty may even be granted release time from teaching in order to pursue such academic activities. Collaborative work can also be the foundation on which letters of recommendation are written for a candidate who is seeking promotion, tenure, or a new job. There is therefore, a symbiotic nature to faculty relationships when it comes to working across disciplines and campuses, as the nature of the work can benefit all members of a group in their professional goals. Journal articles, conference presentations, research, and grant writing serve as professional accomplishments in similar ways across fields. Being a member of a multicampus group that is awarded a prestigious National Science Foundation Grant, for example, looks good on each participant's curriculum vitae.

Disability services staff also work with members of their field who are on other campuses. All parties involved can further the goals of their field and their own professional development by this kind of collaborative work. Again, there is the possibility of conference presentations and publications resulting from this collaborative work and the networking can also serve professional ends. Due to the different nature of the way staff and faculty work is valued, however, including differences in reporting structures and how promotions and salaries are decided, there is far less professional incentive built into current academic systems to encourage collaboration between faculty and staff. Furthermore, while there may be some value given on one's own campus to collaborative work across campus and divisions there is usually nothing built into the system which would either encourage staff on one campus to work with faculty on a different campus, or there is usually even a way built into current systems for staff supervisors to recognize such work as valuable. We will return to this point shortly when we consider staff performance reviews.

Faculty might find a way to develop their work with staff into a journal article, conference presentation, or research project, regardless of if the staff member they have worked with is on their home campus or works for a different institution. The current academic tradition does include an expectation though that each faculty member will be developing their reputation in a specific field and thus, the work a faculty member does typically has to be tied into their own field in order to be most valued in their professional development. While there is [limited] value given to community service, new faculty have very few resources—including time and energy—left to contribute to projects that are not doing double work by also helping to develop their professional reputation within their field. For example, if one teaches writing or literacy, one could volunteer to manage a community literacy project, or if one is in a business field they could volunteer to keep the books for a charity fundraiser. Faculty's professional interests are best served by tying most of their efforts into developing a cohesive professional image.

Of course, the same is true for staff with the biggest difference being that service often has a broader meaning. If an act of service is positively perceived in the community then it by extension reflects well on the school and the school's reputation. While staff can and often do work with faculty, faculty would basically have to be on their home campus and they would need to bring that work back to their home field in order for their efforts to have the greatest professional development impact. One's home campus might value work done with faculty on that same campus; it is much harder though, for the home institution to give value to work done with faculty on other campuses.

Unlike faculty who have a tenure process to go through, staff are more likely to go through a formal "performance review." A performance review usually includes filling out an institutional form that asks specific questions. These reviews, however, tend to ask very job-specific questions related to work carried out within the institution, including: the number of people one supervises; the types of technologies with which one is familiar; the level of secure information to which one has access; and the departments on campus with which one has worked. Unless one is in management there may not even be consideration given for professional presentations or publications as part of the performance review process.[1] If one is a member of staff-management they are more likely to be asked how they are meeting their home institution's goals and what policy developments they've initiated in the past year. While there is some value given to managers presenting and publishing, these are typically considered a smaller part of the staff's role (particularly compared to expectations of faculty). Again, the two groups fill different roles on campus and the expectation is that faculty will do more of the research, writing, and presenting than will staff.

Resource allocation

This is not to suggest that either faculty or staff do only those things which immediately reward them through promotion or retention. The reality is, however, that both groups face such demands on their time and personal resources that taking on work which cannot further their professional careers yet takes time from their professional lives—such activity is not only a lower priority, it may even be frowned upon by their employer. Time, energy, resources, and funding are resources, and resources are expected to be focused on those projects which will either directly or indirectly benefit the institution which employs a person. Employees benefit their institution by developing their own careers and reputations within their fields. Work which cannot be "accounted" for in the traditional ways that are expected, is like volunteer work within the community; while some level of such activity is expected, too much volunteer work can come at the expense of one's career. Too much work outside the "normal" channels can also lead to a perception among managers that an employee is not focused on, or fails to set, appropriate goals.

Remember that we are discussing two separate fields—disability studies and disability services—and work which is perceived to be focused outside one's own field may not be valued by one's home institution.

With the belt tightening that has taken place within university budgets it is challenging, for example, to find financial support or release time to attend conferences within one's primary field. Trying to convince an institution to even partially support attendance at conferences that are outside one's primary field will usually be an uphill battle. Faculty and staff must carefully consider where they will spend their limited time and financial resources when engaging in professional conversations. For some professionals it is not financially feasible to attend conferences which would allow direct dialogue with colleagues in another field, even when it is a neighboring field in disability.

If one wishes to engage in other fields it is often necessary to seek out journals and books which can be read in one's "spare" time. Of course, one cannot engage in a dynamic dialogue in the same way by reading and writing a response, as one can in personal conversation. Conferences thus have value but are not always an economically viable option. And if release time is not given to attend a conference, not only is there the immediate impact of paying out of one's pocket for attending, one must use one's vacation time to do so, time when family and friends may feel they should have more claim on that time versus giving priority to further work projects. Time and personal attention, like money, are finite resources. Faculty and staff tend to find they have so many demands placed on their resources that difficult choices must regularly be made.

Choosing to spend one's resources on disability is in effect choosing to make this work part of one's professional identity; disability studies and disability services are further choices which again narrow one's specialization. Both faculty and staff become known for having areas of special interests and there is a limit to the number of interests a person is professionally able to maintain. Again, trying to be active in too many areas leads to the wider impression that one is ineffective due to a lack of focus and a lack of sustained professional development in any one area. In professional contexts while those of us in the disability fields believe that disability is everyone's concern, other professionals are likely to see disability as our specialization. Our colleagues will tend to view themselves as too involved in their own specializations to become active in our field. Similarly, even others in what I consider "neighboring" fields that share disability concerns, may perceive that it is too much of a stretch to become involved in one more field. There is still considerable work to be done demonstrating the potential overlap between concerns and projects that each field has independently developed and focused on; not everyone will perceive that the potential coalitions which can be formed are worth the expenditure of resources that such collaborations will require. Educating ourselves is necessary and the lack of shared education and thus collaborative goals is another obstacle to creating coalitions in the first place. This leads us to the next obstacle to collaborations between the fields—a lack of shared professional space where such education and discussions can take place.

Lack of shared professional space

Currently both fields, that is, disability services and disability studies, have their own conferences, publications, and professional organizations. And while some individuals attend and participate in both conferences and have membership in both groups, they are for all the reasons already discussed, by far in the minority. There is no current professional space that is in effect co-owned by the fields, either in print or in physical meetings. Again, the reasons for this should now be clearer. Lacking such shared professional space is an obstacle to greater dialogue, work, and cooperation between the fields; there is also a lack of shared space for education to take place regarding the potential for coalition forming.

Consider, for example that staff people are at best usually supported to attend one conference a year (not all receive this support) and that they are most likely to use that support to attend a conference in their immediate, rather than a neighboring field. The same is true for faculty. There is enough professional emphasis on presentations and publications, however, that faculty may be able to personally justify paying at least partially out of pocket to attend additional conferences that allow them opportunities to develop their curriculum vitae and projects. Staff will likely not have this same option, in part because they do not have the same release time from work to attend conferences.

Another difference between workloads and expectations which impact times when the two groups of professionals are even available to build cooperative projects is reflected in their contract expectations. Most staff are expected to be on campus for 12 month contracts, while faculty contracts typically are for 9 months; faculty in theory at least have the remaining three months available for research, writing, and if needed travel to further these causes. This allows faculty more flexibility in where they will be physically located while staff are typically expected to be physically present on campus. This is another way in which faculty tend to have more freedom to attend conferences outside their primary field, while staff will typically have release time from work only to attend conferences within their primary field.

Due to these differences in job expectation, the way resources are allocated both personally and professionally, and a lack of shared professional space it should now be clearer why it is neither easy nor natural for collaboration between the fields to take place. Given these challenges and the different roles that each field is responsible for filling on an academic campus it thus becomes logical to ask what is to be gained that would make the effort and expense worth taking on? What do the fields themselves gain by forming coalitions which lead to shared projects and goals? What do people with disabilities stand to gain and how is society impacted by collaborative efforts—or is something lost socially when there is a lack of coalition forming between fields? In what follows we will consider first what the fields have to gain from collaboration and then consider what the social payoff might be to collaborative efforts.

A difference that matters

One of my philosophy professors used to be very fond of the saying, "In order to be a difference, it has to make a difference." The first time any poor student dared to respond with a blank look this professor would launch into a mini-lecture pointing out that there are many differences in the world and that difference in and of itself is not notable (he was a pragmatic ethicist). Differences counted when they amounted to disparity. For example, if you choose to have vanilla ice cream, and I choose chocolate, that is a difference. The difference, at least from an ethical/philosophical viewpoint, does not matter—it carries no weight.

Let us consider the possibility though that we both have vanilla ice cream. You're happy because you wanted vanilla anyway. I, however, wanted chocolate but was denied my choice because chocolate ice cream is being hoarded by a special interest group and additionally—you were offered a choice while I was not. You still chose vanilla but I didn't have a real choice because I was only offered vanilla. Now we're talking about a difference that makes a difference. Two people are eating vanilla ice cream but only one of those people was given a choice about which kind of ice cream they would eat. If this were a philosophy class we could now have a very spirited discussion about equity and society and is a society "fair enough" where everyone has at least vanilla ice cream or ought everyone have at least the choice of whether or not they have chocolate? Or is this a "first world" concern, where we argue about access to ice cream while others are worried about access to clean water? (It can be very difficult to keep a philosophy class on-task with a discussion because metaphors can be taken in so many unintended directions rather quickly.)

The point for the purpose of our current line of inquiry—the fact that disability services and disability studies are both on campus and have projects related to academics, students, and society yet have almost no overlap or shared projects—is this a difference that makes a difference? Does this reality impact anyone or change anything? A slightly different way of asking this question is to consider: What projects become possible if the two fields deliberately combine efforts?

Contentious claim

While both fields make use of theory and practice, I argue that neither field uses theory or practice in balance. Obviously some may find this a controversial claim and it will be necessary to bear with me as I develop my argument. My contention is that at the moment disability studies tends to favor the meta view of disability, while disability services tends to favor a normative view of what actually ought to be done in daily practices.[2] This is particularly true within the contexts of academic settings regarding the respective role each field has within the institution. I am not claiming that either field is focused on the one to the exclusion of the other, far from it; I am suggesting the fields have taken on different emphases due in large part to the different roles they fulfill on campus and expectations within academic institutions of the respective roles of each field.

In volume 34.2 (2014) of *Disability Studies Quarterly (DSQ)*, Brewer and Brueggemann (2014) report on their analysis of *DSQ* during the publication years of 2000–2012. Within this article the authors note:

> We might also view the presence of words like *rhetoric, communication, language,* and *reflections* [emphasis original] as an indication that scholars are interested in issues of representing oneself and others. How we do (and should or shouldn't) talk about disability is as much a part of Disability Studies as topics like the ADA, new media, and poetry.

They note that *DSQ* continues to publish personal essays and poems about the experiences of people with disabilities, making a point to include first-person narratives. These narratives provide crucial reminders of both the importance of the work that disability studies does and the areas in which further work is still needed. I argue that this work often takes on a meta viewpoint, in part because this is the nature of what academics are expected to do. One must include not just the theory which underlies one's work, one must tie their project into the larger field and show why what is proposed makes a difference.

The point I am illustrating is reflected in this observation from the same article, "For example, the terms *new*, *paradigm*, and *models* suggest that contributors to *DSQ* during this time had a self-awareness that their writing was proposing a new way of looking at disability issues" [emphasis original]. It is also noteworthy for the point I am making that while an analysis of keywords that appear for articles from *DSQ* includes the words, "identity," "policy," "representation," and "social," the keyword "practice" does not occur. I maintain that this is due to an academic-research tendency toward looking at meta issues of disability, a viewpoint faculty have traditionally been encouraged to take.

In Volume 27.1 (Spring 2014) of the *Journal of Postsecondary Education and Disability* (JPED) the longest published journal of the disability services field, editor David R. Parker stops to reflect on 30 years of publication and notes that:

> As the Journal launches its 30th year, we celebrate the evolution of knowledge, beliefs, and practices regarding postsecondary education and individuals with disabilities. One important example of that growth is the refinement of evidence based practices that measure what we know about students with non-apparent disabilities and the impact of our work with them (p. 3).

JPED issues are typically heavily focused on practices; in this same issue there was one article with a meta focus—"An Initial Investigation into the Role of Stereotype Threat in the Test Performance of College Students with Learning Disabilities"; five articles that looked at practice and applications; and one article that was a combination study/first-person account of postsecondary education experience from a self-identified person with a disability, "(dis)Ability and Postsecondary Education: One Woman's Experience" (Meyers et al., 2014).

The primary emphasis of each field is also reflected in the annual conferences held by the Society for Disability Studies (SDS) and the Association on Higher Education and Disability® (AHEAD), respectively. *SDS June 26–29, 2013, in Orlando, Florida,* had the theme "(Re)Creating Our Lived Realities" and the conference announcement states,

...this year's conference theme seeks to explore the myriad ways in which we work to (de)construct the various realities in our lives. Whether through laws, policies, militaries, language, rituals and customs, or the many decisions we make in our daily lives, we are constantly transforming and being transformed by the built material, social, and cultural environment(s) around us" ("Past Conferences").

AHEAD 2013 in Baltimore, Maryland, July 8–13, had the theme "Challenging and Changing Disability Perspectives" and the conference announcement states,

> Explore how the disability climate is changing and how these changes are influencing practices and outcomes in the higher education disability environment ("Welcome").

Notice the difference in focus between the large picture, meta issues, and focus on implementation at a normative level. In the next chapter I will suggest that there is something to be learned on each side by hearing one another when focus tends to be somewhat different between the two fields; this is another reason that coalition forming and collaborative projects have something to gain from deliberate interactions. Using examples from a journal article from *DSQ* and a journal article from *JPED* I will illustrate with specific examples of what the fields might gain from a more intentional dialogue. Dialogue ideally will lead to the forming of coalitions and consideration of the question, what potential do such coalitions have?

Chapter 6: Thought points

- ▶ What do I consider to be two of the most significant potential obstacles that would keep the fields of disability studies and disability services from taking part in productive dialogue that might lead to productive coalitions which could speak about issues of disability? How would I suggest overcoming these potential obstacles?
- ▶ When I approach a subject to conduct research, do I tend to focus on larger meta issues like the social systems that led to a context, or do I tend to focus on normative issues like how to change the practices in specific types of contexts? How do—or can—I explain why I have this preference? Do I have an example of a time when I successfully bridged the two in one project?

▸ If I am a participant in one of these fields, what questions would I be interested in asking participants in the other field? After visiting the web site where past conference topics are listed, what is an example of a topic I would like to learn more about and what intrigues me about this topic?

SDS "Preliminary Program" 2013
   http://www.disstudies.org/conferences/orlando-2013/preliminary-program
   AHEAD "Concurrent Sessions" 2013
   https://www.ahead.org/conferences/2013/concurrent.

Notes

1 My doctoral dissertation included an analysis of staff performance reviews as part of a literacy project, *Preparing Writing Centers and Tutors for Literacy Mediation for Working Class Campus-Staff.*
2 For a fuller discussion of how I define "meta" and "normative", see Chapter 7.

7
Potential Impact of Intentional Interaction and Coalition Forming

Abstract: *This chapter defines how Meta and Normative are being used and applied to the respective fields and then applies these concepts to an article from DSQ and one from JPED to show specific examples of how each field frames specific concerns; how does the conversation within and between fields change when each field adopts something of the viewpoint of the other? What questions grow out of dialogue that are less likely to be produced by the fields working independently?*

Keywords: changing social focus; creating shared professional space; disability coalitions

Oslund, Christy M. *Disability Services and Disability Studies in Higher Education: History, Contexts, and Social Impacts.* New York: Palgrave MacMillan, 2015.
DOI: 10.1057/9781137502445.0009.

The ivory tower. This common social reference to academia is a way of pointing out what socially is perceived as a difference between what happens on university campuses and what happens in "the real world." Not everyone seems to recognize that an academic campus is not located outside real life but just one more part of life. Aside from birth, death, and taxes, few experiences in life are universal; not all of us will compete in a Mr. Universe contest, or spend a season crab-fishing in Alaska, or milking cows on a dairy farm—not everyone will spend time on a college campus. But all of these experiences are part of some people's real lives and statistically, far more of us will attend college/university than will take part in contests of physique or be employed in any single specialized job.

The interactions between larger society and college campuses also can result in some significant long-term social changes that would not have happened as/when they did if not for activity that grew out from campus life and activity. What happens on campus—the discussions and ideas that are generated here—are both a reflection of what happens in the wider world and in turn impact social movement, thought, language, and behavior in the wider world. When a group of people gather for the express purpose of sharing knowledge it is logical that they are likely to be the source of new ways of seeing and responding to events surrounding them.

College campuses in the U.S. were a critical point of social action and conscious-raising, for example, during the civil rights movement; globally, college students are some of the people most likely to challenge the social status quo. As Mike Oliver (2009), an academic and activist from the UK notes,

> It was during the 1970s that women were beginning to reject male accounts of their experiences and black people were vehemently denying the accuracy of white descriptions of what it was like to be black. This questioning has reverberations through the academic world, calling into question the whole notion of objectivity and bringing subjectivity onto the academic agenda. (p. 16)

As was earlier discussed, the disabilities rights movement grew in significant ways as a result of organizing, activism, and networking that began on campuses and then spread out into the community. Particularly in an age of growing social media use, where actions and activities from campus are immediately shared with a potentially global audience, life on campus is also simultaneously life in the larger social world. In the chapter, "The Cyber-Propelled Egyptian Revolution and the De/Construction of Ethos" Samaa Gamie, for example, demonstrates how two Facebook pages begun by young people, acted as political catalysts and became "the voice and face of the youth movement that ignited the Egyptian revolution" (Oliver, 2009, p. 316). Social media expedites the sharing of a range of ideas including those which will prove to be initiators of social change, and young people on college campuses are some of the most fluent social media users, even if at times they have much to learn about the impact of their social media use (Folk and Apostle, 2013). What happens both in the classroom and on the wider campus is mutually influenced by the larger community and in turn influences far beyond the campus boarders.

Campus life has also been a reflection of the larger social response to people with disabilities. When societies are reluctant to create accessible processes and places then too are their colleges, which are often small mirrors of larger social attitudes. When educational institutions are at their best however, they can be the starting points for positive social change, with affects that ripple out into the communities around them, in turn influencing larger social adjustments. Colleges can both replicate and reinforce the status quo and they can challenge dominant social policies; many campuses have both types of activity going on at the same time.

This flow of ideas and information leads me to the next consideration: What impact does it have on campus and in the wider community when disability services and disability studies have so little overlap? We will then consider, as mentioned at the end of the last chapter, what the two fields might have to gain from pursing deliberate coalition with shared projects.

Meta and normative

In previous sections we established that faculty and thus the disability studies field is encouraged to focus on the meta level of disability while staff and thus the disability services field is encouraged to focus on the normative level. Before building any further on this claim, let us consider in more detail the difference between meta and normative as being used here; again we note a difference because it impacts the approach and outcome of something—in this case the relationship of the respective fields to disability.

[Reminder—we have already located disability in society as opposed to in individuals, therefore a field's relationship to disability also implies relationships within society.]

I am using *meta* herein to refer to *the big picture view* including analysis of how systems function and how these functions and interactions lead to certain outcomes. I recently came upon what may now be my favorite definition of how we use "meta" to refer to higher order considerations. From the *Online Etymology Dictionary* by Douglas Harper (2014):

> Third sense [of meta], "higher than, transcending, overarching, dealing with the most fundamental matters of," is due to misinterpretation of metaphysics as "science of that which transcends the physical." This has led to a prodigious erroneous extension in modern usage, with meta- affixed to the names of other sciences and disciplines, especially in the academic jargon of literary criticism, which affixes it to just about anything that moves and much that doesn't.[1]

A used and living language is one more system that undergoes redesign; while Mr. Harper may find it objectionable that meta has become "corrupted" nonetheless it is increasingly used to refer to overarching considerations. In the case of disability studies, some examples of what I would identify as meta-studies would include considering how historical usage of the word "disabled" has been morphed by time, place, and social group; how legal systems interact with those identified as disabled; how the label of disabled may in the future be impacted by modern applications of technology; how disability is portrayed in media—these are just some examples of the meta focus prevalent in disability studies.

Normative as used herein is influenced by the concept of normative ethics, which is not the same as "normal"; in ethics, *normative indicates how things ought to be*. Disability services tends to focus on not just practices as they are but on what the best possible practices ought to be. The normative view of disability is the act of both identifying what best [service/social] practices would be and then working toward implementing these practices and the necessary supporting policies. In the case of disability services, some examples of what I would identify as normative-studies or normative-practices would include reviewing the process necessary within a school for a student to receive accommodations and potentially modifying the process to be more student-centered; evaluating a program's current evaluation tools; evaluation/education of how to make online learning more accessible—these are just some examples of the normative focus prevalent in disability services.

To restate: I am not suggesting that either field uses either focus to the exclusion of the other. My argument is that the very nature of their respective roles within institutions influences the domination in one field of a meta focus and in the other of a normative focus. Does it not make sense, however, that when two fields have become so specialized yet continue to share some centralized concerns, that these fields might benefit from dialogue and deliberate coalition building?

One might counter, of course, that we have just established that these two specialized fields have specific roles within institutions and there is in fact little need for overlap and shared interest between them as a result. Ironically perhaps, I would acknowledge that this point has some merit and as a result we will return to this consideration in detail in *Chapter 8*. For now, let us focus on the effects the current state of semi-isolation (with little overlap) and specialized focus are having.

Balancing perspectives through dialogue

In this section I will use an article from *DSQ* and then one from *JPED* to illustrate how a conversation begun in one field can potentially change if it became a topic of discussion between fields. In *Chapter 8* we will then consider some possible shared goals that a coalition between the two fields might have, or be supportive of, if they more deliberately work together.

A thoughtful and well-written piece by Soldatic and Grech appeared in *DSQ 34.2*. "Transnationalising Disability Studies: Rights, Justice and Impairment" asks some very difficult questions: What is the impact on those disabled through violence and war when "disability" is being naturalized, even celebrated? The authors point out that in a global arena there is a "tendency to assume that human rights and citizenship rights are mutually constitutive" (Vol. 34.2). They then point out that not all people enjoy citizenship as part of a stable nation, while others have actually become disabled as a result of violence carried out on behalf of their government. What is the impact on disenfranchised people who are disabled through aggression when those of us who are in more privileged circumstances claim disability is normal or that disability is part of our identity, perhaps even fundamental to our culture? The authors also note that there is currently often no satisfactory response for those who have been displaced by war and violence which results in disability, because so many nations exclude the disabled in their immigration policies, while the home state of a person may be the entity responsible for acts of violence against the individual, making repatriation ill-advised.

It is natural that research and scholarly work will raise questions, and that some questions raised may not be answerable. I do not mean to imply for a moment that part of the work that disability studies and disability services will accomplish by creating arenas of overlap is to "answer" each other's questions. Actually, in dialogue they may discover further questions which will be equally complicated. This in fact may be a significant part of what will come out of their dialogue—new questions and intricacies added to standing queries. Research and normative practices both grow, however, from questions asked.

From personal narratives (Anderson et al., 2014; Linton, 2006; Meyers et al., 2014) to research which indicates the personal and academic cost of the stigma both historically and still attached to disability (Lightner et al., 2012; Rimmerman, 2013; Stiker, 1997), *both disability services and disability studies* in northern countries do tend to argue for normalizing disability. As northern activists argue for normalization of disability, how will both fields respond to concerns such as those raised by Soldatic and Grech? How, for example, do I as a disabled person who is also an academic respond when, even as I am in the midst of arguing that there ought to be no stigma to claiming an identity of disabled, I am reminded that I am also privileged to be in a position to voice any claims, and to speak out and reach an audience? What will it mean going forward to recognize that I am both privileged and stigmatized? How will the tension inherent in my position be reflected in my future projects; will those topics which I address be impacted by these questions and if so, how?

I would suggest that participants in both fields can be reminded by Soldatic and Grech's article that we are largely benefiting from some form of power, be it the opportunity to seek a degree, teaching, researching, or even having access to income or resources which allow one to read books like this—we do tend to enjoy privileges. I think, for example, of a show I was listening to on National Public Radio which said that increasingly poverty in the U.S. means a poverty of hope and future; this version of poverty may include owning a vehicle and television (Fessler, 2014). In a nation where parents may have economically reached heights their children are less likely to reach, "gifts" of automobiles and technology mean someone can own a smart phone yet have no food in their cupboard or have a car to drive to a job which does not pay a living wage.

In other countries, poverty might mean 13 people living in a room; a lack of safe drinking water; the possibility of being sold into slavery. Is it possible for either disability studies or disability services to speak across the chasm of lived experience or are we only deluding ourselves to think that we can speak of disability concerns on a global scale? Are those of us in powerful nations speaking of disability in a way that further problematizes life for people with disabilities who are disenfranchised? That might be a fairly meta-question. A more normative question might be: Granted that a student in the U.S., Canada, England, or Australia might not have known the brutality of life that a war refugee has, will this knowledge impact how we work with this student's story of personal trauma and stigmatization? Should the one impact the other? Do we have responsibilities as educators and service providers to raise awareness of how much more people with disabilities in other geographic locations struggle, or is it even possible to compare personal struggle? How can we discuss these very different experiences of what it is to be disabled, in the same space and what happens if we do not discuss these very different experiences of being and becoming disabled?

As both educators and service providers, we can also enter into discussions about what are our primary responsibilities; do we ever need to make choices between the students we work with and wider issues of disability? Either way, how do these potentially conflicting concerns impact what we teach and those situations which we hold up for people to learn from? And what does it imply when we hold up examples of rape and torture as acts of disablement to people who have perhaps been born disabled or acquired disability in a less traumatic way? How in our own work do we balance these very different kinds of stories? Should the meta-knowledge of disability caused by violence impact my interactions with the student sitting in my office at any given moment talking about their personal experience of disability? How can I assist the student or coworker who questions their own story of disability when they are faced with stories that seem "more horrific" or in disagreements, if within a discussion someone in the north argues that "local" disability does not count in the same way as this "more horrific" disability; can disabilities count "equally?" And here's a meta-question with a normative impact—how do we educate people that disability ought not to be more or less horrible, that disability is not a matter of equity between types of disability? Can we together design a specific application (a class) which looks at both disability inflicted through violence and disability present from birth; what would the pedagogical goals of such a class be? These are the kinds of questions that impact both disability studies and disability services. Having these conversations might also lead to identifying potential goals for social changes which would then be pursued.

JPED 26.1 included the article, "Assessing the Impact of ADHD Coaching Services on University Students' Learning Skills, Self-Regulation, and Well-Being" by Field et al. (2013) which compared results when students living with attention deficit hyperactivity disorder (ADHD) were provided academic "coaching" support while a control group of ADHD students continued to work independent of structured coaching. One of the primary goals of this study was to provide research-based evidence to show what, if any, impact coaching has on students with ADHD; previous studies have indicated that students with learning disabilities and ADHD benefited from coaching.

In this particular study, carried out with students from 8, 4-year universities and 2 community colleges, coaching was not provided on campus in person; students and their coaches talked by phone once a week and could check in with each other by phone or e-mail as needed during the week. Knowledge and skill areas covered by the study included executive functioning and impacts on students' focus, time management, and anxiety management. Those students who received coaching demonstrated positive outcomes in all areas including "statistically significant higher executive functioning" (Field et al., 2013, p. 77) both compared to when they began the program and compared to the control group, that is, the group which had no regular coach meeting. Coaching was provided for six months.

How ought the growing evidence that individual academic support improves the retention and academic progress rates of students be impacting how we structure our classrooms and our disability services programs? How should both schools and society be adapting to the changing nature of our students and young people, when young people increasingly require types of teaching and support which are not commonly available? What roles should disability studies and disability services be taking on: impacting the social perception of what it means to learn and to collaborate; impacting academic perceptions of what counts as individual effort vs. "plagiarism"; beginning conversations and educational efforts on and off campus about differences in learning?

What projects might be possible if combined efforts are made between fields to further study the impact of academic coaching, personal mentoring, and the role of encouragement on rates of success? Is increased success due to mentoring/coaching limited to school; how do workplaces change if the young people entering the workforce benefit from more deliberate mentoring than previous generations may have required? What roles can specialists within fields fill that spreads these ideas beyond their classroom, office, or institution? Individually, if we analyze how we currently spend our time with students and compare that time with the students' need for one-on-one support, is there any indication that we may need to change how we are spending our time? Institutionally, how much individual attention or mentoring is available for students and are policies in place to adjust these numbers in the face of increasing need?

The articles and questions we have just considered are only two examples of how taking a subject from one field into another can complicate work and research on a personal and professional level. It would seem that perhaps the greatest gain to be made from more deliberately creating spaces of dialogue between disability services and disability studies is that questions for individuals and for each field will result which otherwise would not have and again, it is from these questions that new areas of research, service, and practice will grow, as well as clearer goals formed as part of a coalition agenda, which would in turn lead to different social action and education. If we can create opportunities and shared professional spaces for dialogue then we can develop projects that otherwise will not develop. Practitioners within specialized fields also bring a different point of view to a conversation so that when ideas and research are more widely shared, further innovations will be sparked. The biggest question remains—how will we create these shared spaces for dialogue given obstacles of limited resources including time and funding?

Chapter 7: Thought points

These thought points require you to choose a primary field to identify with—either disability services or disability studies.

- ▸ What would you say to convince a reluctant member of your own field that they should consider spending some of their limited

resources exploring the "other" field? Make the most persuasive argument you can and provide a specific example of a project your fields might collaborate on.
▸ If you were talking to members of the other field, what is to you the most exciting work in your field that you would like to share with them? What project might you propose working on together and what role could you fill in that project? What would you like to learn about from their perspective?
▸ A number of potential questions and areas of further research were raised in this chapter. Which to you would make an interesting area of further exploration and research? What questions of your own would you like to explore in relation to this topic and how might you go about beginning this exploration?
▸ If you know someone working in the neighboring disability field consider if you have ever discussed with this person what they value most about their field. Are you aware of any projects or research they have worked on? What about your own work you have discussed with this person? Can you think of a potential collaborative project that the two of you might consider working on together?

Note

1   http://www.etymonline.com/index.php?term=meta-

8
Building Collaborative Efforts through Coalitions

Abstract: *This chapter explores the potential of a coalition between the fields when specific collaborative projects are taken on. It first considers some of the collaborative work currently being done and then moves on to consider where there is pressing need for current coalition action. For example, currently on campuses students and employees with mental illness are perceived as the "dangerous disabled" even though they are more likely to be the victims rather than perpetrators of crime. This is just one example of the need for combined voices/actions that will change both the campus and larger social climate, yet is an area where there is no concerted effort being made between the fields to deliberately educate and advocate.*

Keywords: collaborative coalition goals; meta v. normative practices; reframing disability discussions

Oslund, Christy M. *Disability Services and Disability Studies in Higher Education: History, Contexts, and Social Impacts.* New York: Palgrave MacMillan, 2015.
DOI: 10.1057/9781137502445.0010.

When was the last time you attended a conference presentation, lecture, or public talk which excited you? This of course sounds like a question meant to set up the idea that all too often we attend presentations that are not exciting; actually I am thinking of the opposite point—can you recall being excited by an idea that framed something in a new way or presented something new-to-you? Focus on a specific exciting idea. I would speculate that the excitement you experienced was tied to one of several reasons: The topic was directly related to an area or idea that interests you; the topic had application to something you are personally working on or would be interested in working on; the outcome of future work on the topic could lead to change that interests you.

Now think about how much follow-up you have done in pursuit of this exciting idea. Are you currently working on anything related to it—taking a class or planning to offer a class on the topic, writing a paper, working on a proposal for a presentation? Are you in collaboration with others who are working on a contingent idea/project? I am working toward making a twofold point here. First, we are revisiting an argument made earlier; each of us has limited resources of both time and money and must choose very specific projects to work on, out of many exciting possible projects available to work on. Second, whatever projects we do choose to work on generally are tied not just to our field but our particular specialization within that field; no matter how much an idea excites us, if we cannot find a way to tie it into the work we are paid to do, or the area we are studying and specializing in, we probably cannot justify the time and energy necessary to significantly develop something new. Collaborative ideas can be very exciting but it can become a time-consuming process of creative thinking and labor to find a way to tie an exciting idea into our own existent work. This is true for students as well as for working professionals in either field—we all resource limitations and must choose where we will "spend" our finite hours in a day.

As exciting then as the idea of creating greater collaboration and dialogue between disability studies and disability services may sound (at least for some of us) does the very specialized nature of our respective work on campus make the reality of shared dialogue and work improbable? Is this the type of idea that might raise some interest at a conference but prove problematic when it comes to actual implementation?

A philosophy professor I knew used to teach that the correct answer to most questions was "yes and no." Yes, this dialogue is complicated and in some specific contexts may not even be currently possible. No, it is

DOI: 10.1057/9781137502445.0010

not universally impossible or beyond inception; it will doubtless take small steps to move our fields down the path toward greater sharing of ideas and work. To my mind an obviously better set of questions is thus: Are there examples of collaboration already taking place; where are some of the current openings for dialogue and shared projects; if we build a coalition between these fields what concerns might our united voices address; and what are the potential social impacts of these shared goals? It is also worth noting some of the complications to be mindful of. In creating new space for dialogue how do we avoid creating an even more specialized and restricted or exclusive area of practice? Arguably, northern academic concerns are already moving away from concerns experienced by southern, disenfranchised people with disability. Being mindful of this can make a difference in those projects which we choose. How can we mindfully spend our limited resources of energy and time so that they have the most beneficial social and academic impact?

Specific collaborative examples

I will begin with what I witnessed at the 2013 AHEAD conference in Baltimore. AHEAD's July conference is an annual gathering of disability services professionals and much of what is discussed there regards normative practices—how things are currently done and the direction that best practices ought to be taking. Taking part in and leading some of these presentations was Tammy Berberi, the president of the Society for Disability Studies (SDS) (Berberi, 2013). Throughout the conference Dr. Berberi was one of a handful of people present actively promoting greater dialogue between the fields of disability studies and disability services. On behalf of the SDS she invited everyone present at AHEAD to attend the following year's SDS conference and otherwise encouraged greater dialogue between the two groups of professionals. In her presentation, "What's in a Name" she also challenged disability service providers to consider the impact on students when so many of the service-offices have "disability" in their title, yet 75% of students who qualify for service do not self-identify as disabled. This is an example of the kind of cross-field posing of questions which becomes possible when professionals make a point of intentionally crossing fields.

Kimberly Tanner (2013), the Access Office Director for Valdosta State University provided information and examples from her own work of collaboration with a disability studies professor at Valdosta State. This example suggests a step that professionals in both fields can adopt as a first step—cross-campus collaboration. And this is perhaps the next logical and most feasible step for the majority of professionals in both fields to adopt.

In order to provide some other examples of the type of collaborative work that is happening on other campuses, I will also use several examples of collaboration from my own work. On my current campus there is no professor specializing in disability studies and therefore I do not have access to on-campus collaboration with another "disability" specialist. There is however, a Humanities department and within that department there is a specialization of teaching Technical Communication. I have worked as a "client" for technical communication classes asking groups of students to look around our campus with a different lens than they are used to seeing through and to assist me in finding ways in which our environment including classes, spaces, and processes can be made more accessible. This collaboration between professors, students, and I has resulted in exchanges of ideas as well as more tangible products such as a new map showing all the accessible washrooms on the main campus, a documentary of campus life from the perspective of a student who transports herself by scooter, and installation of accessible doors and signage in multiple locations across campus. Despite my penchant for philosophy I have a great fondness for idea exchanges and knowledge acquisition which sometimes lead to practical applications such as these. Physical outcomes are not always practical but sometimes—particularly for young people who enjoy seeing results from their work—this can be a happy marriage of concepts, goals, and concrete results.

To use a less physical example however, I have also had opportunities to collaborate with a professor from the Social Science Department who teaches an American Government class with the underlying theme of institutions and norms. I have enjoyed spirited discussions with her classes about the development of government policies like the Americans with Disabilities Act. The liveliest discussions arise when we talk about service animals, therapy animals, and accessibility. The students are fascinated by the roles animals can play outside of family-pet and have shown a willingness to provide greater social access to assistance animals as well as beginning to understand the harm it does when people try to game the system by pretending their dog is a service animal when it is not. These are very small pieces, simple examples of how we can work where we are to increase collaborative projects and dialogues which at least open topics for discussion. While anecdotal in nature I can witness changes in attitudes and behavior in colleagues and students as we continue to make opportunities for shared work. The point is, while I look forward to the day when there will be a professor who specializes in disability studies on campus, and would love to see our campus develop at a minimum a disability studies minor, in the meantime I continue to look for the work and collaborations I can achieve given our current context.

Opportunities for dialogue

The obstacles that were previously shown to complicate an increased dialogue between the two fields show that most of these obstacles exist for work that would take place between professionals in disability studies and disability services *on different campuses*. Most of these complications do not apply, however, to projects which would grow from greater collaboration amongst professionals employed by the same institution. Perhaps the greatest obstacles to on-campus collaborative work all grow from issues of time: time for additional work; time to meet with colleagues who have different obligations regarding when they will be on campus; time to develop new ways of looking at our shared educational mission. We are most likely to be able to make choices which reallocate our time when we become determined that a type of work, or a specific project, is worthy enough that we will make it a priority, *and* the project has support from our home institution because it works in concert with local priorities.

While it might seem too great a jump for most of us to immediately begin attending conferences outside our specialization, that is, to spend our resources at the other field's gatherings, we can make time to identify one or two projects on our home campus which have the potential for collaboration with multiple stakeholders. We can at the very least make time to host initial meetings and conversations which begin the work of exploring the possibilities of dialogue—and learning more about each other's work. This is the type of cooperative effort that is usually favored by one's employer. The managers of academic institutions see a shared mandate of education, retention, and building a favorable ethos for a campus—all of which can be furthered by a growth in collaborative efforts that share a goal of improving social conditions (on and off campus) for people with disabilities. In fact, given our current social climate, administrators across campus will prove open to discussions which are shown to share a goal of increasing diversity on campus, improving student retention, and improving the larger social climate for diverse populations. In effect, we are in a position to promote the argument that disability is both complex and a significant part of diversity; to continue to point out that discussions of diversity have often overlooked the component of disability which ought to be included and that as long as exclusion of disability continues when considering mandates to increase diversity, we will continue to academically lose students.

The topic of diversity in academics traditionally focusing on ethnicity is a prime example of a topic that the two fields could speak more loudly about if a coalition were formed with shared topics and goals. Before we move on to consider social goals, however, let us consider another way that we can become more informed about the field that is not our primary field.

Self-educating about the "other" field

Journals are the lifeblood of information about current trends, debates, and new developments in any academic or professional field. While maintaining subscriptions and keeping up with the reading are further investments of resources, these tend to be more manageable investments than would be attending a national conference. In Chapter 7 there was mention made of a journal available in each field: *Disability Studies Quarterly (DSQ)* and T*he Journal of Postsecondary Education and Disability (JPED)*. These journals are included in membership when one joins the respective professional networks, The Society for Disability Studies, and the Association on Higher Education and Disability®. One can also subscribe to the journals without joining either association, or request that one's school library obtain an institutional subscription to the journals.

Other nations also have publications, including online journals known as "zines," as well as archives available on the web. The University of Leeds, Center for Disability Studies, maintains a valuable online archive of publications in the disability studies field at http://disability-studies.leeds.ac.uk/library/. The site is deliberately accessible and intended to be used by "disabled people, student, and scholars" who wish to learn more or conduct research in the disability studies area. Another valuable site, *Disability Studies: Online Resources for a Growing Field*, is hosted by the American Library Association (2010) and lists resources available including zines, radio shows, online exhibitions, associations, and annotated bibliographies.

One can also learn more about active discussions within each field by joining one or more "listserves"—a type of e-mail subscription where one receives an e-mail whenever any member of the list sends it to the "list." Lists often develop around special interests, and there are also lists within each field, and within one's home nation. By joining a broader field list such as each field has, one will on occasion read about a specialized list that is being formed to discuss more focused interests, which will include specific topics, and sometimes regional concerns. Lists can be time consuming to keep abreast of; however, they are a way to keep an "ear open" to the ongoing concerns and most recent discussions within a field; unlike journal subscriptions lists tend to cost time rather than money and they can point one toward further topics of reading/research, as well as educational material.

There are ways, in other words, of becoming familiar with the concerns of a specialized field without attending the field's conferences or even without attending classes. Of course, a class, a discussion group, a presentation, a webinar—these all inform/teach in different ways and to different degrees. The larger point is simply that there is more than one way to begin to become familiar with the concerns of each field in general and more specifically to begin thinking about possible points that a coalition might initially agree on, some shared goals that might be a starting place to work from. Coalitions are made up of groups that may not share exactly the same agenda; however, the groups can work together to bring greater attention—and in the case of these specific fields—broader social education to mutually agreed upon topics. Voices also become stronger when there are more of them joined together calling for the same action, such as a specific social change; these changes are needed not just in the wider community but also on academic campuses. Coalition forming is a way to bring people with common concerns together to voice shared calls for action.

Why collaboration and coalitions matter

Bernice Johnson Reagon spoke about the use of coalitions, explaining that when a group is ready to step outside their own "barred room" into the wider world a coalition allows groups with some overlapping concerns to have a stronger voice when they speak together. Reagon cautions that if a group remains isolated it is like keeping themselves in a locked room and that eventually larger forces will clear house; staying in the locked room has simply made the group an easy target for removal since they're all in one confined space. She also warns that coalitions are not about being comfortable but about surviving. The more global our world becomes, the less possible it is to remain isolated, "There is nowhere you can go and only be with people who are like you. It's over. Give it up" (1983/2000, p. 344). Reagon provides sound reasons for forming coalitions, including the opportunity to gain strength in numbers. Her underlying theme that isolation from difference is no longer possible is a theme that a disabilities coalition could adapt; we can agree that both campus and larger social groups need to realize, understand, and better prepare for the reality that disability can no longer be isolated, kept in a room where the bars are on the outside holding the people with disabilities within the room. The members of a coalition can together speak about the need to be more socially prepared for the presence of people with disabilities not just in classrooms but also in work and all other social contexts.

I cannot help but remind myself of the slogan started by Queer Nation, "We're here, we're queer, get used to it." People with disabilities are not going away, they are going to continue to seek access to the same spaces and opportunities that other members of society are given access to. Not surprisingly, Crip Theory has been influenced by Queer Theory and Feminist Theory, challenging social norms and the way, as Kafer says, "the kinds of spaces we imagine often determine the kinds of bodies/minds that can inhabit these spaces" (2013, p. 152). One does not have to identify as a particular type of theorist, however, to take part in a coalition which questions the kinds of bodies and minds that society is currently used to imagining in public and professional spaces. The classes that Kafer teaches, for example, are more often identified as "feminist studies" rather than "disability studies" and this is another benefit of collaborative efforts that grow out of strong coalitions—we can educate and speak about social injustice that impacts a range of marginalized people (p. 151). This is one of the reasons that on some campuses disability support services have begun to align themselves with centers for diversity and inclusion. Those of us who make up "diversity" have in common the experience of being excluded from mainstream social acceptance in a range of social spaces and activities. There are many types of body which have not traditionally been imagined as belonging in academics, in specific social positions, or in leadership roles either on or off the academic campus. Disability studies and disability services ought to be working more cohesively in helping society to reimage the types of bodies which are able to occupy public spaces and roles.

This returns us to a point previously raised: The actions, concerns, and ideas of society can be influenced and affected by those of us who work in academic settings, and by those of us who take classes, who read books and articles, who are willing to have difficult conversations, and who choose to not close their minds to new ways of thinking and new ways of seeing the society in which they participate. We can each act as agents of change. I am suggesting that coalitions are strongest when they are made up of academics and citizens, the disenfranchised and the powerful, the voices of personal experience and the voices offering meta theory for why society ought not to continue on a path it is on.

From personal experience and conversations with colleagues I know, for example, that it is still far too common for institutions and individuals to take the paternalistic view that X class/activity/area of study is too difficult/dangerous/unrealistic for anyone with Y disability.

Instead of allowing individuals with disabilities to find their own success and failure as other citizens do, too often social forces try and stand in the way; we continue to "protect" which in effect is simple exclusion of those we perceive to not belong where they wish to try and go.

Not all who read this work, for example, will be spending their professional lives in academia. The question for those working in other fields becomes: How can I take what I know/learn about people, about disabilities, about social contexts, about exclusion—how can I take this knowledge into my work and community and what projects and collaborative efforts can I be part of which will help promote inclusion of greater diversity where I work, live, and play?

Touching lives as we collaborate

Thanks to the widespread use of digital media I recently heard Naval Admiral William H. McRaven's 2014 commencement speech to the University of Texas at Austin. Admiral McRaven pointed out that if in a lifetime you are able to touch just ten people's lives and make a meaningful difference, and each of those people touch ten people's lives to make a difference etc. there is the potential for exponential outreach from that humble starting point. One of the amazing things about working or studying in academia is that we have the opportunity to interact with hundreds, even thousands of others who are interested in learning and often interested in having an impact on society. One of the incredible things about our current digital age is that each of us has the capacity to impact the spread of news and ideas—we can each have influence on the way our social groups enact values; we can choose to make our spaces, conversations, groups, and thoughts more or less inclusive, albeit having more inclusive thinking is perhaps the hardest work any people can challenge themselves to do. Ideas, however, are only a starting place and until we put our principles into action our ideas themselves are not as powerful as they will be when they lead to action.

Perhaps in fact, being more collaborative minded regarding connections outside our specialized field is the most significant impact any of us interested in changing contexts related to disability can bring to our social interactions. Nonetheless, I cannot shake the conviction that we will gain something more when the deliberate sharing of projects between disability studies and disability services becomes more commonplace. I also believe that the wider the dialogue the more likely it will spread beyond the space of campuses and classrooms, and the less time this sharing will take. Coalitions are strongest when they include people who live and work both inside and outside the academic context. A strong coalition is more than individual voices and individual actions. A coalition requires that individuals join in identifying set shared goals, decide on some shared projects even if those projects are then carried out in more local ways in numerous locations.

Potential coalition goals: a starting place

One possible goal of a coalition might well include rethinking the current divisions present in academics which make collaborative work so challenging. Interdisciplinary study is not valued by all academic institutions and even on those campuses where it is valued, the focus remains on faculty. How could the system redesign so that collaborative efforts between faculty and staff become more valued?

It is also significant that academic institutions continue to mirror social views of disability being a problem located within individual bodies. As Price (2011) points out in *Mad at School*, in academics we still focus on the individual student and the medically defined limitations of their bodies and minds. Mental illness, for example, is part of the human condition and as was previously mentioned, historically mental illness did not socially mean that a person could not also be a student, teacher, or participant in events. It is much more recently (and as Price indicates, often in reaction to school shootings) that there is both a larger social and academic knee-jerk reaction, that someone with mental illness should be excluded from participation, from holding roles as a student or teacher. There is fear that people with mental illness will harm those around them based on the perceived potential harm that those who are mentally ill are feared to represent. People with mental illness are more likely to be the victims rather than perpetrators of violent crimes but society currently views mental illness as a violent disability.

Access is another potential coalition subject of education and action. In *The Question of Access*, Titchkosky explains that access "needs to be understood—as a complex form of perception that organizes sociopolitical relations between people in social space" and then poses the question, "Now, what if, like access, we treat disability as a way of perceiving and orientating to the world rather than conceiving of it as an individual functional limitation?" (2011, p. 4). The fields of Disability Studies and Disability Services might agree on the theoretical concept that disability could be conceived of as a way of orientating to the world; however, larger society requires more education before this becomes a broader held view. Price's point, that people with mental illness are not welcomed in academic settings, also shows that socially and academically we within academic settings are just as guilty of still employing the practice of identifying individual bodies based on their medical diagnosis, particularly when it comes to the potential and limits we perceive the minds of others to hold. This certainly seems like an area where there is a strong need for a coalition of voices to join in educating both the academy and larger society; if the disability fields are not working together to problematize social views of mental illness and current views of people with mental disabilities, then there certainly is a large gap between the theories espoused and the practices being lived. If we hesitate to share classroom, campus, shopping, or other public spaces with people with mental disabilities, how can we expect our larger societies to become more accessible? If we deny a segment of the population access to education and social space based on their disability, how can we claim to be working from a social justice model? And even if we as individuals do promote greater accessibility, how much more could we be accomplishing, how much more effective could our advocacy be, if we were part of a coalition that had many members working toward similar goals?

Coalitions need not be limited to disability studies and disability services; an advocate or person with disabilities may not identify with either field, and a student might take one class in a field and go on to work in something completely unrelated. As Reagon points out, coalitions gain strength when diverse people work together toward shared goals. I would also argue that given the recursive nature of beliefs and behaviors within society and formal educational settings, it does seem increasingly odd that there are not more active collaborations between the two specific fields of disability studies and disability services; if we do not work together to challenge ignorance, stereotypes, and urban myths then we in effect affirm the dominate social stigmas. There certainly is a great deal of room for coalition building between fields and intentional identification of shared goals and projects which we can together work toward. A coalition cannot form, however, if we do not step out of our separate rooms and clarify and act toward achieving our shared goals.

Chapter 8: Thought points

- Can you identify any collaborative efforts in your local community which appear to be the result of a coalition of interest groups working together to address a local need? Research how the collaborative effort began and what has been necessary to keep the group going (i.e., fund-raising; volunteers; space donated or rented, etc.).
- List three specific issues related to disability that you are currently aware of (these could be local, national, or international). Using preliminary research if necessary, suggest one potential coalition discussion/project you could propose that would address each of these issues. Identify a specific goal for each collaboration. Which of these three could you most feasibly become an active participant in and why?
- Having read and hopefully discussed the ideas contained herein, have any new ideas been sparked for you? Take time to make note of these ideas, then mark your calendar and remind yourself to revisit these ideas in four weeks; at that point see if the ideas that

struck you as noteworthy four weeks ago have resulted in any action. Ask yourself if new thoughts are leading to new projects and if not, why not? What is standing between you and coalition forming and collaborative projects? If you believe something is important are you taking actions to live this value in the world?

Works Cited

Act 103 of 1937. State of Michigan. Michigan Legislative Website. Viewed at http://www.legislature.mi.gov, November 25, 2013.

AHEAD. (1996). "AHEAD Code of Ethics." Viewed at http://www.ahead.org/learn/resources, November 30, 2013.

AHEAD. (2012). "Featured Presentations and Events." *Association on Higher Education and Disability*®. Viewed at http://www.ahead.org/conferences/2012/awards_lunch, November 25, 2013.

AHEAD. (2013). "About AHEAD." *Association on Higher Education and Disability*®. Viewed at http://www.ahead.org/about, November 25, 2013.

AHEAD. (2013). "Welcome from Conference Chairs." Viewed at https://www.ahead.org/conferences/2013, May 6, 2014.

American Library Association. (2010). "Disability Studies: Online Resources for a Growing Field." Karen Moss Ed. Viewed at http://crln.acrl.org/content/71/5/252.full, July 25, 2014.

Anderson, D., Anderson, D., and Hudson-Weems, C. (2014). *The Rosa Parks of the Disabled Movement, Plantation Politics*. Bloomington: Author House.

Berberi, T. (2013). "What's in a Name." *AHEAD Concurrent Session 8.3*. July 12, 2013.

Biblica Inc. (2011). *Holy Bible*. New International Version. Grand Rapids: Zondervan.

Black, K. (1996). *A Healing Homiletic: Preaching and Disability*. Nashville: Abingdon Press.

Works Cited

Bogdan, R. (1990). *Freak Show: Presenting Human Oddities for Amusement and Profit*. Chicago: University of Chicago Press.

Bragg, R. A. and Wagner, M. K. (1968). "Can Deprivation be Justified?" *Hospital and Community Psychiatry* 19.7, 53–54.

Brewer, E. and Brueggemann, B. J. (2014). "The View from *DSQ*." *DSQ*. 34.2, Viewed at http://dsq-sds.org/article/view/4258/3598, May 5, 2014.

Buck V. Bell. (1927). United States Supreme Court.

Buell, J., Stoddard, P., and Charlton, J. I. (1998). *Nothing About Us Without Us: Disability Oppression and Empowerment*. Berkley: University of California Press.

Charlton, J. I. (2000). *Nothing About Us Without Us: Disability Oppression and Empowerment*. Berkeley: University of California Press.

Descartes, R. (1641). *Meditations on First Philosophy*. Trans. Donald A. Cress, 4th ed. 1999. Indianapolis: Hackett Publishing.

Fessler, P. (2014). "The Changing Picture Of Poverty: Hard Work Is 'Just Not Enough.'" *War on Poverty, 50 Years Later*. National Public Radio, aired July 5, 2014.

Ferguson, P. M. and Nusbaum, E. (2012). "Disability Studies: What is it and What Difference Does it Make?" *Research & Practice for Persons with Severe Disabilities*. 37.2, 70–80.

Field, S., Parker, D. R., Sawilowsky, S., and Rolands, L. (2013). "Assessing the Impact of ADHD Coaching Services on University Students' Learning Skills, Self-Regulation, and Well- Being." *Journal of Postsecondary Education*. 26.1, 67–81.

Finkelstein, V. (1980). *Attitudes and Disabled People*. World Rehabilitation Fund: International Exchange of Information in Rehabilitation. Monograph #5, New York.

Folk, M. and Apostle, S. (Eds) (2013). "Preface." M. Folk and S. Apostle. *Online Credibility and Digital Ethos: Evaluating Computer-Mediated Communication*. Hershey: IGI Global, xvii–xix.

Galton, F. (1883). *Inquiries into Human Faculty and Its Development*. New York: The Macmillan Company.

Galton, F. (1904). "Distribution of Success of Natural Ability Among the Kinsfolk of Fellows of the Royal Society." *Nature*. 70.1815, 354–356.

Gammie, S. (2013). "The Cyber-Propelled Egyptian Revolution and the De/Construction of Ethos." Eds. M. Folk, S. Apostle. *Online Credibility and Digital Ethos: Evaluating Computer-Mediated Communication*. Hershey: IGI Global, 316–330.

Gladwell, M. (2008). *Outliers: The Story of Success.* New York: Little, Brown, and Company.

Goddard, H. H. (1912). *The Kallikak Family.* New York: The Macmillan Company.

Goffman, E. (1986). *Stigma: Notes on the Management of Spoiled Identity.* New York: Touchstone.

Goodey, C. F. (2011). *A History of Intelligence and Intellectual Disability; The Shaping of Psychology in Early Modern Europe.* Farnham: Ashgate Publishing.

Harper, D. (2014). "Meta." *Online Etymology Dictionary.* Viewed at http://www.etymonline.com/index.php?term=meta-, May 9, 2014.

"History: Twenty-Five Years of Progress in Educating Children with Disabilities Through IDEA." (updated 2007). *Special Education and Rehabilitation Services.* U.S. Department of Education. Viewed at http://www2.ed.gov/policy/speced/leg/idea/history.html, March 26, 2014.

Horner, R. D. (1980). "The Effects of an Environmental "Enrichment" Program on the Behavior of Institutionalized Profoundly Retarded Children." *Journal of Applied Behavior Analysis.* 13.3, 473–491.

Hume, D. (1777). *An Enquiry Concerning Human Understanding.* Ed. Eric Steinberg, 2nd ed. (1993). Indianapolis: Hackett Publishing.

Johnson, H. M. (2003). "Unspeakable Conversations." *The New York Times.* February 16, 2003. Viewed at http://www.nytimes.com/2003/02/16/magazine/unspeakable-conversations.html, February 6, 2014.

Kafer, A. (2013). *Feminist, Queer, Crip.* Bloomington: Indiana University Press.

Kant, I. (1785). *Groundwork of the Metaphysics of Morals.* Trans. T.K. Abbott (2013). Cedar Lake, MI: ReadaClassic.

Kittay, E. F. (2010). "The Personal is Philosophical is Political." Eds. Kittay and Carlson. *Cognitive Disability and its Challenge to Moral Philosophy.* West Sussex: Wiley-Blackwell, 393–413.

Kuhn, T. (1962). *The Structure of Scientific Revolutions.* Chicago: University of Chicago Press.

Lane, W. L. (1974). *The New International Commentary on the New Testament: The Gospel of Mark.* Grand Rapids: Eerdmans Publishing Group.

Lightner, K. L., Kipps-Vaughan, D., Schulte, T., and Trice, A.D. (2012). "Reasons University Students with a Learning Disability Wait to Seek Disability Services." *Journal of Postsecondary Education.* 25.2, 159–177.

Linton, S. (2006). *My Body Politic*. Ann Arbor: University of Michigan Press.

Lipsky, D. K. and Gartner, A. (1997). *Inclusion and School Reform: Transforming America's Classrooms*. Baltimore: Paul H. Brooks Publishing Co.

McRaven, W. H. (2014). "Ten Life Lessons from a Navy Seal." Posted on *LifeBuzz*. Viewed at http://www.lifebuzz.com/10-lessons-from-navy-seal/#!RY5IL, May 25, 2014.

Meyers, M., MacDonald, J. E., Jacquard, S., and Macneil, M. (2014). "(dis)Ability and Postsecondary Education: One Woman's Experience". *Journal of Postsecondary Education*. 27.1, 73–87.

The National Archives. (2001). *The Royal Earlswood Hospital, Formerly the Earlswood Asylum, Redhill, Records* (392). British Crown: Surrey History Center. Viewed at http://www.nationalarchives.gov.uk/a2a/records.aspx?cat=176-392#0, November 25, 2013.

NCD, "About Us." *National Council on Disability*. Viewed at http://www.ncd.gov/about, November 25, 2013.

Nielsen, K. E. (2012). *A Disability History of the United States*. Boston: Beacon Press.

Oliver, M. (2009). *Understanding Disability: From Theory to Practice (2nd Ed.)*. New York: Palgrave Macmillan.

Oslund, C. M. (2011). *Preparing Writing Centers and Tutors for Literacy Mediation for Working Class Campus-Staff*. Michigan Technological University Digital Commons Viewed at http://digitalcommons.mtu.edu/cgi/viewcontent.cgi?article=1092&context=etds, April 23, 2014.

Price, M. (2011). *Mad at School: Rhetorics of Mental Disability and Academic Life*. Ann Arbor: University of Michigan Press.

Polioplace (2011). "Judith Ellen Heumann." *Post-Polio Heath International*. Viewed at http://www.polioplace.org/people/judith-e-heumann, November 25, 2013.

Quinn, G. (2013). "Foreword." Ed. Arie Rimmerman. *Social Inclusion of People with Disabilities: National and International Perspectives*. Cambridge: Cambridge University Press.

Reagon, B. J. (1983/2000). "Coalition Politics." *Home Girls: A Black Feminist Anthology*. 2nd Edition. New Brunswick: Rutgers University Press, 343–356.

The Richard III Society (2013). Viewed at http://www.richardiii.net/, November 25, 2013.

Roberts, E. V. (1980). "The Emergence of the Disabled Rights Movement." Text of speech, *Online Archive of California*. Viewed at http://www.oac.cdlib.org/view?docId=hb6m3nb1nw&brand=oac4&chunk.id=meta, March 24, 2014.

Roets, G., Adams, M., and Van Hoove, G. (2006). "Challenging the monologue about silent sterilization: implications for self-advocacy." *British Journal of Learning Disabilities*. 34.3, 167–174.

Ryerson University. (2014). "School of Disability Studies Viewed at http://www.ryerson.ca/ds/, March 6, 2014.

Schweik, S. (2009). *The Ugly Laws: Disability in Public*. New York: New York University Press.

Shakespeare, T. (2013). *Disability Rights and Wrongs Revisited*. New York: Routledge.

Shakespeare, W. (1993) "The Life and Death of Richard III." Ed. Jeremy Hylton. *The Complete Works of William Shakespeare*. Viewed at http://shakespeare.mit.edu/, November 26, 2013.

Shapiro, J. P. (1993). *No Pity: People with Disabilities Forging a New Civil Rights Movement*. New York: Times Books.

Shaw, G. B. (1912). *Pygmalion*.

Siebers, T. (2008). *Disability Theory*. Ann Arbor: University of Michigan Press.

The Sterilization Act of 1924. (May 20, 1924). Virginia General Assembly, *Acts of Assembly*, p. 569.

Society for Disability Studies. "Mission and History." Viewed at http://www.disstudies.org/about/mission-and-history, February 2, 2014.

Society for Disability Studies. (2013). "Past Conferences." Viewed at http://www.disstudies.org/annual-conferences/past-conferences, May 6, 2014.

Soldatic, K. and Grech, S. (2014). "Transnationalising Disability Studies: Rights, Justice and Impairment." *Disability Studies Quarterly*. Viewed at http://dsq-sds.org/article/view/4249, May 1, 2014 (34.2).

Stiker, H. J. (1997). *A History of Disability*. Trans. W. Sayers. Ann Arbor: University of Michigan Press.

Syracuse University, *The Center on Human Policy, Law, and Disability Studies*. "Academic Programs in Disability Studies." S. J. Tayler and R. Zubal-Ruggieri. "What is Disability Studies." Viewed at http://disabilitystudies.syr.edu/what/whatis.aspx, February 2, 2014.

Syracuse University, *The College of Law*. "International and Comparative Disability Law Web Resources," (2010). Viewed at http://www.law.syr.

edu/library/electronic-resources/legal-research- guides/humanrights. aspx, July 22, 2014.

Tanner, K. (2013). "Out of the Box II: Provocative Conversations to Challenge Seasoned Professionals and Push Our Thinking Beyond the Status Quo." *AHEAD: Preconference Institute.* July 9, 2013.

Titchkosky, T. (2011). *The Question of Access: Disability, Space, Meaning.* Toronto: University of Toronto Press.

UC Hastings. (2013). "Paul Grossman, Adjunct Faculty." *University of California Hastings College of The Law.* Viewed at http://www.uchastings.edu/academics/faculty/adjunct/grossman/index.php, November 25, 2013.

University of Leeds, Center for Disability Studies (2014). *The Disability Archive UK.* Viewed at http://disability-studies.leeds.ac.uk/library/, July 25, 2014.

Winship, A. E. (1900). *Jukes-Edwards: A Study in Education and Heredity.* Harrisburg: R.L. Meyers & Co.

Wright, N. T. (1998). "Foreword to the New Edition," Ed. Marcus J. Borg. *Conflicts, Holiness, and Politics in the Teachings of Jesus.* New York: Continuum International Publishing Group, ix–xxiv.

Index

ablebodiedness, 29
ADHD, 101
Alison Kafer, 81
Allan, 47
Andrew Reed, 43
Architectural Barriers Act of 1968, 55
Association on Higher Education and Disability® AHEAD, 56
Attitudes and Disabled People, 73
Australian Disability Clearing House on Education and Training ADCET, 57

Bearnice Johnson Reagon, 81
Bragg &Wagner, 48
Buck v. Bell, 34
Bureau of Jewish Education, 36, 118

Canadian Association of Disability Service Providers in Post-secondary Education CADSPPE, 57
Center for Independent Living, 54
C.F. Goodey, 38
Chang and Eng, 31
Charles Stratton, 31

coalition, 81, 82, 84, 88, 89, 92, 96, 98, 102, 106, 109, 110, 111, 113–16
Colin Barnes, 76
collaborative work, 84, 107, 108, 113
conjoined twins, 31
Crip Theory, 4, 111

David Hume, 40
Descartes, 39
disability, 2
Disability Rights Movement, 49
disability service specialist DSS, 17, 59
disability services, 5, 8, 83
disability studies, 5, 8, 9, 30, 70, 71, 75–9, 83, 90, 91, 98, 106, 109
disabled people, 4
disablement, 100
DSQ
   Disability Studies Quarterly, 90

Ed Roberts, 54
Education of all Handicapped Children Act EHA, 48
equity, 89
Erving Goffman, 27
eugenics, 33, 38

European Disability Forum
   EDF, 57
Eva Feder Kittay, 42

faculty, 8, 9
Ferguson and Nusbaum, 76
freak shows, 30
Fundamental Principles of Disability, 72

gender equity, 81
George Bernard Shaw, 41
Gerard Quinn, 53

Harriet McBryde Johnson, 43
Hebrew Scriptures, 22
Henry H. Goddard, 34
Horner, 48

IDEA
   Individuals with Disabilities Education Act, 48
Identity, 3
Immanuel Kant
   Kant, 41
Individual Education Plan
   IEP, 49
individual impairment, 75
Individuals with Disabilities Education Act
   IDEA, 47
intellectual and developmental disabilities
   IDD, 34, 38
interdisciplinary, 77

James I. Charlton, 46
Jeff McMahan, 42
Jo Anne Simon, 57
Joan Leon, 55
Joseph P. Shapiro, 54
Journal of Postsecondary Education and Disability, 91
Judy Heumann, 54
Jukes, 34

Kallikak Family, 34
Kathy Black, 26
Kim E. Nielsen, 44

limited resources, 102, 103, 105, 106
Lipsky and Gartner, 49
Little People UK, 3

Malcolm Gladwell, 47
Mallett and Slater, 4
Marilyn Bartlett, 57
medical model, 24
meta, 90, 97
Mike Oliver, 73, 95
miracles, 29, 30

National Council on Disability Education NCD, 56
National Science Foundation NSF, 12
normative, 90, 92, 97
normative practices, 99
N.T. Wright, 24

Office of Civil Rights (OCR), 60
Old Testament, 22

Paul Grossman, 57
people with disabilities, 4
performance review, 86
Peter Singer, 42
Physical barriers, 53
poverty, 100
practice, 2, 40, 46, 49, 62, 90, 91, 102, 106, 114
progeria, 31
P.T. Barnum, 30, 32
public education, 71

re-designs, 6
Rehabilitation Act of 1973, 55, 56
resource allocation, 86
Restricted Growth Association, 3
rhetorical appeals, 39

Richard III, 28
Rimmerman, 53
Robert Bogdan, 30
Roets, 35
Royal Earlswood Hospital, 43
Ryerson University, 78

Samaa Gamie, 96
Samuel Gridley Howe, 45
Section for the Study of Chronic Illness, Impairment, and Disability, 75
Self-awareness, 51, 118
service provider, 17
Sir Francis Galton, 33
Snyder and Mitchell, 79
social context, 75
social media, 96
Society for Disability Studies (SDS), 75
special education, 46, 48, 58
staff, 8, 12
Standards and Performance Indicators AHEAD, 63
stigma, 4, 20, 27, 46, 48, 99

stigmatized, 17, 27, 28, 29, 31, 47, 49, 50, 80, 99
Susan Schweik, 32
Syracuse University, 68, 71, 76

theory, 63, 74, 88, 90, 91, 112
Thomas Kuhn, 63
Thought Points, 18, 35, 50, 67, 81, 92, 102, 115
Tobin Siebers, 3, 36, 118
Tom Shakespeare, 4, 74
Tom Thumb. *See* Charles Stratton

ugly laws, 32
Union of the Physically Impaired Against Segregation UPIAS, 71
universally designed education, 17
University of Washington, 78
U.S. Department of Education, 47

Vic Finkelstein, 72, 73

William L. Lane, 25
World Health Organization (WHO), 4
World Institute on Disability, 55

GPSR Compliance

The European Union's (EU) General Product Safety Regulation (GPSR) is a set of rules that requires consumer products to be safe and our obligations to ensure this.

If you have any concerns about our products, you can contact us on

ProductSafety@springernature.com

In case Publisher is established outside the EU, the EU authorized representative is:

Springer Nature Customer Service Center GmbH
Europaplatz 3
69115 Heidelberg, Germany